THE PERFECT MEDICINE

BRODIE
RAMIN, M.D.

THE PERFECT MEDICINE

How Running Makes Us Healthier and Happier

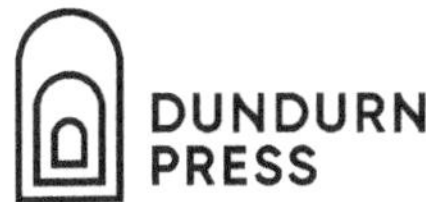

Publisher: Scott Fraser | Acquiring editor: Kathryn Lane | Editor: Dominic Farrell
Cover and interior designer: Laura Boyle
Cover image: Unsplash.com/Jeremy Lapak
Printer: Marquis Book Printing Inc.

Library and Archives Canada Cataloguing in Publication

Title: The perfect medicine : how running makes us healthier and happier / Brodie Ramin, M.D.
Names: Ramin, Brodie, 1982- author.
Description: Includes bibliographical references and index.
Identifiers: Canadiana (print) 20210167513 | Canadiana (ebook) 2021016770X | ISBN 9781459748200 (softcover) | ISBN 9781459748217 (PDF) | ISBN 9781459748224 (EPUB)
Subjects: LCSH: Running—Health aspects. | LCSH: Running—Physiological aspects. | LCSH: Running—Psychological aspects.
Classification: LCC GV1061 .R36 2021 | DDC 613.7/172—dc23

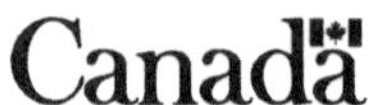

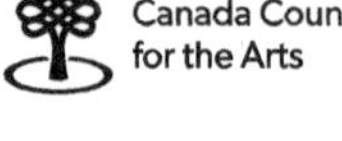

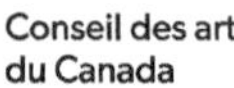

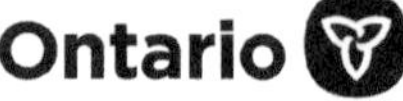

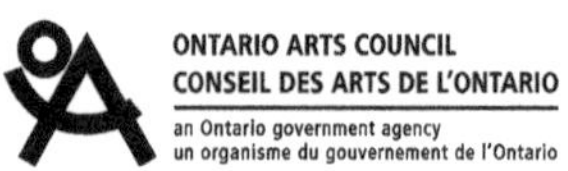

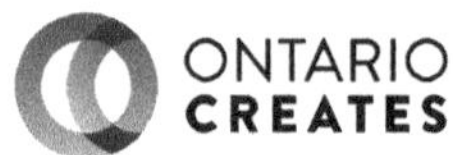

We acknowledge the support of the Canada Council for the Arts and the Ontario Arts Council for our publishing program. We also acknowledge the financial support of the Government of Ontario, through the Ontario Book Publishing Tax Credit and Ontario Creates, and the Government of Canada.

Printed and bound in Canada.

Dundurn Press
1382 Queen Street East
Toronto, Ontario, Canada M4L 1C9
dundurn.com, @dundurnpress

To my family, who always urge me on when the road seems long

To my family, who always urge me on when the road seems long

CONTENTS

PREFACE

I awake with a start as the scream of an ambulance fills the night air. Then come the words from the hospital public announcement system: "Anesthesia to the emergency room. Stat." People are running; urgent calls for medication and oxygen echo toward me. The halls teem with human bodies urgently pushing forward.

We run for different reasons throughout our lives. Children run for the purest pleasure, chasing or being chased, thrilling at the hunt. We run toward a finish line, toward safety.

Someone has been stabbed in the abdomen; he's just a teenager, a boy. Outside, there are three police cars with their lights flashing. More doctors are called stat to the emergency department. *Stat* comes from the Latin for *immediately.* We want things immediately; our patients need blood or medicine immediately.

So much of modern life is done on the run. We run to aid those in need. In ancient Rome, running was a metaphor for life. Philo of Alexandria observed that it is "rare for God to allow a man to run life's race from start to finish without stumbling or falling."

The boy dies during the night, and as I step out of the hospital the next morning, it hits me. With all our stat orders and the power of modern biomedicine, we couldn't save him. I walk home along the icy sidewalk. The wind blows rippling spirals through the snow. I am at the end of my primary care residency and about to start another year of training in HIV and addiction medicine. It's winter in Ottawa, and my life has taken many turns to bring me to this hospital to do this job.

Ten years earlier I was beginning my undergraduate degree in political science, and I went to a birthday party in a dimly lit restaurant. A recent graduate from the same program told me that she had decided to change fields and go into medicine. As she explained her rationale — a desire to work with people, to be a scientist, to understand the human body — I knew what I had to do. I ran home, dropped my courses, and signed up for the pre-medical sciences. She was my guide, and I would follow her lead into medicine.

"Chance favours the prepared mind," Louis Pasteur said, in reference to his own discoveries. Sometimes you don't realize a major truth until some act of chance pulls the curtains open to reveal something you knew all along or pushes you to do something that was waiting inside. So it was with medicine, and with running. When the time came for me to become a runner, a chance discussion with my brother set me on course to live and breathe running, to revel in its richness and see into its science.

I now run almost every day and practise a blend of addiction medicine and primary care in Ottawa. I've written about the opioid epidemic and the machinations of Big Pharma. I know there are medications that save lives, but I also know that medicine and public health is more than pills and injections. I want to explore the power of exercise to improve health. And as I approach the end of my thirties and see my forties looming over the horizon, I want to learn how to be a better runner, how to keep my mind and body supple, how to ride the wave of aging as gracefully as possible. It's time for me to write about running.

I once heard an author tell an interviewer that you should only write a book if you can't stop yourself from doing so, if the words are racing out. I feel that compulsion about running — I just can't help from putting my shoes on, heading out the door, and putting one foot in front of the other. I've become fascinated by running and what it means to be a runner. I've also been inspired by the growing scientific evidence that tells us how to run faster and farther and which reveals that running is a powerful way to achieve better physical and mental health. I wrote this book because I couldn't stop the words from racing out.

What's your first memory of running? I am in the second grade and it's a bright day. Everyone is chasing me. I see a swell of children and I feel the absolute importance of escaping the tide, bursting through an opening, evading their hands. I thrill at the rush of speed my legs give me. I am fast and I love the feeling. Roger Bannister, the English physician who became the first man to run a mile in less than four minutes, describes standing barefoot on firm, dry sand as a child and feeling overwhelmed by beauty. In his memoir, *Twin Tracks*, he writes:

> For once, there was nothing to detract from this feeling of closeness to nature. In this supreme moment I leapt in sheer joy and started to run. I was startled and frightened by the tremendous excitement that so few steps could create.... I was running now, and a fresh rhythm entered my body.... I discovered a new unity with nature. I had found a new source of power — a source I never dreamt existed.

My usual run starts at home. I leave my front door and run slowly down the sidewalk. I turn right, and in a minute, I am running along the Rideau Canal, a man-made waterway that bisects Ottawa after flowing two hundred kilometres down the landscape from Lake Ontario. I run along the canal and cross under the Bronson Street Bridge. With a sharp inhalation, I leave my crowded neighbourhood of old brick homes and arrive at Dow's Lake, which stretches in front of me, the arboretum and the city's Experimental Farm beyond it. I run along the lake then up a small incline where, in the summer, men open locks designed to lift or lower boats along their way. To my left is Carleton University, where my father studied journalism and economics in the 1970s.

I've run here so many times that the normally hard distinctions between seasons in Canada blend in my mind. In the winter the canal is frozen solid, and I will run down a flight of rubber stairs to join thousands of skaters gliding up and down the length of the frozen expanse. I stay on the snowy covering just to the side of the cleared ice and focus on my breathing and my feet, looking for cracks and lumps in the ice.

Sometimes I run along the canal path when it is dark, with only the glow of a crescent moon to light my way through fallen leaves. Sometimes it is midsummer, with a full sun overhead. Sometimes it is six in the morning and my children are just stirring awake on a spring day.

I reach a bay where the Rideau River meets the canal and a dam controls the flow of water. One night in March I see a boat on the river with glaring lights illuminating its path. I have never seen this before. I stop to watch as what looks like a steamboat paddle-turns and lifts the craft onto the still-solid ice of the river before the ice gives way and the front of the ship comes down. It is breaking the ice in anticipation of the coming thaw.

I feel awed watching this mechanical beast work through the night. The feeling mixes with the other physical and emotional products of running: heat, euphoria, breathlessness, calm. Afterward, I sit on my back porch, looking out at the night, thinking about what I have seen, my breath slowing, my pulse returning to normal, the swirl of neurochemicals surging through my brain, priming me to run again.

More than ten million people in North America run at least one hundred days a year.[1] Over the last thousand years, runners were hunters, messengers, and champions. We evolved to run in the African savannah. Runners functioned as the nervous system of the Incan empire, with messengers connecting the hinterland to the seat of power. In Germany, runners spread news and personal letters until the 1700s, when the development of the postal service replaced them. We invented a sedentary world then discovered jogging. We told ourselves stories about great runners then created the marathon to celebrate the journey of a messenger.

One cold December 31, I ran in Ottawa's Resolution Run, a 5K race through the freezing darkness of New Year's Eve. Hundreds of runners lined up for the last race of the year. The turnaround point was a few metres from my house, and when I reached it, I wanted to give up and sprint for the warmth of home. Thirty minutes of standing around outside before the race had left us all so cold. It was well below freezing, and within a few minutes of the starting gun, the moisture had formed solid ice on my eyebrows and eyelashes. I tried to blink the ice away as I picked my way through the crowd in the darkness.

There were no timing chips or kilometre markers. The zipper on the running jacket I got with the race package had already broken. What kind of race was this? It made me glad to be done with the old year; the new one would have to be better than this. Next year, I would work on running my fastest 10K time yet. I would run my first trail race, and I would run my first marathon. I couldn't wait to get started.

1 BEGINNING TO RUN

I was born in the hospital to which I would return thirty years later as a medical resident. One of the last snowfalls of the year blanketed the city as my parents carried me into our small house across the street from Manor Park. Two years later my family moved to Port-au-Prince, Haiti's capital city. My father's work in international development and my mother's job as a teacher kept us moving every couple of years, always leaving a place just as it became familiar. In Haiti my brothers and I practically lived outdoors. We chased each other through the house and clambered on the orange-tiled roof. We were sunburned and covered in mud from the ravine at the bottom of our garden. When my father came home from work, my brothers and I would follow him outside onto the concrete porch, and while he lifted weights, we played at exercise.

We would drive in our red Toyota Tercel the ninety kilometres to Jacmel, a beach town on the southern coast of the island. The short distance would take hours thudding over the muddy half-built roads. The ocean at Jacmel was fierce. I remember the feeling of being swept under the water as a wave crashed over me. My small body was gripped by the undertow as I struggled to my feet, and I learned to respect the ocean. We spent the nights in small concrete huts just off the beach listening to the sound of crashing waves.

My brother Sascha was born while we lived in Haiti. My mother travelled to Ottawa to deliver him then returned when he was only a few weeks old. I remember the volume of paraphernalia she brought back with her; it seemed like so much equipment for such a small person. He would grow into a tall and lean athlete, unbeatable on a bike, able to run at a blistering pace long before I took up the sport. My older brother, Alex, has a heavier build — he lifted weights and learned judo — but he would also go on to be a dedicated and fast runner.

In 1988 we moved to Bali. It was a paradise, and my parents granted me the freedom to explore. From the age of seven I was given free rein — I headed out on my bike and explored the rice paddies and surrounding villages. I flew kites and ventured down to the beach, and one day I stopped in a field under a perfect blue sky and learned to tie my shoelaces. Perhaps I didn't venture far, but I felt I could traverse the island in complete safety.

The world seemed so big back then. In 1991, during the time of the Gulf War, I sat in class at Bali International School looking at an issue of *Time* magazine that detailed the types of jets and missiles deployed against Saddam Hussein's regime. I felt a vague sense of unease knowing there was a war somewhere else in the world, but we did not have CNN, so I had only a blurry concept of what this meant.

My family moved to Tanzania when I was eight, and there I ran and raced my way through elementary school. I remember racing down the small hill next to our classroom in a cluster of boys and girls. We practised doing front flips by launching into handstands then flipping onto our feet. I felt that this was an incredible feat, but others went even further. Two of my friends — a pair of twin boys — could run into a front flip without touching their hands to the ground. Amazing us even more, they could do backflips. They were daredevils. I stuck to front flips.

In Tanzania we travelled frequently, roaming ever farther from our home in the capital city of Dar es Salaam. My parents and two brothers bundled into our white Land Cruiser and ventured north toward Kenya. We explored the Serengeti, Ngorongoro Crater, and Mount Kilimanjaro. We passed through the towns of Moshi and Arusha, which I would return to twenty years later as a medical student. One day we turned off the main road, and the tires started to churn up dust around us. My father kept driving, but with almost no visibility. The dust started to come in through the ventilation system, and I could taste the grit like sandpaper. All of a sudden sunlight streamed in the windows. We had broken through and arrived at Olduvai Gorge.

Presumably, my parents had told me about our destination earlier that morning, but it would have meant nothing to me. How could they have explained the earliest beginnings of humanity to a ten-year-old? Even today my most vivid memories of the day are driving through that fountain of sand and dirt and the darkness inside the car. But I also remember seeing a monolith of dirt and rock projecting out of the landscape with variegated strata, which to my mind represented the layers of time. *Homo habilis* occupied the site from nearly two million years ago followed by *Homo erectus*, and in the last seventeen thousand years came *Homo sapiens*. That day at Olduvai Gorge has come back to me countless times as I have studied biology, medicine, and the history of our species.

Olduvai Gorge embedded in me a deep and early appreciation of the fact that modern humans are the product of millions of years of evolution in the African savannah. We often hear that humans have "Stone Age brains." Although the societies in which humans live are unimaginably different than those of our ancestors, our bodies have not changed much. As a result we find it difficult to cope with the modern world. Anxiety, for example, is said to be the consequence of primitive instincts that lead us to be always on the lookout for threats; obesity is caused by our urge to consume high fat and sweet sources of nourishment. In Olduvai Gorge the fear of threats and the compulsion to consume as much high-energy food as possible were positive adaptations; indeed, they were essential for survival. In contemporary Shanghai or New York, they are not only less useful, but they are causing epidemics of suffering and leading to premature death.

While the Stone Age brain explanation for the problems suffered by modern humans is often oversimplified, it is true that we have to accept our brains and bodies as they are and design a world that optimizes human health and well-being within the scope of those limitations. Unfortunately, we have not been very successful at doing so. As a result, most people today, adults and children, do not eat properly, nor do most get the exercise and connection with nature we all need and crave.

Living and travelling in East Africa showed me that nature is a wonder to behold; I learned, too, that it is a primal force to be respected. I remember cowering in the back seat while we drove across a flat grassy plain in Tarangire Park in northern Tanzania surrounded by hundreds of elephants. I glanced out of the window to see the herds marching serenely by. On an earlier trip to Kenya, an angry female elephant had charged us, protecting her calf from our Land Cruiser. Humans are masters of the world, but we are also fragile, anxious bipeds who do well to run for cover when confronted by a threat.

Another year we travelled south to the Selous, which was, at that time, an enormous and relatively pristine nature reserve nearly devoid of human habitation. We boarded a small motorboat that spluttered down the Rufiji River toward a pod of hippos. I felt acutely exposed in the small boat as we drifted amid these ton beasts, any one of which could have crushed our little vessel in an instant if instinct had urged them on to such an act.

That first day in Olduvai Gorge was like so many others, as I walked amid the baobab trees, boulders, and coarse vegetation. As my brothers and I played tag or raced or climbed, we were expressing the same basic urges to move and play felt by our ancient ancestors there. Every time I have returned to East Africa since my childhood, I have felt as if I have come home. Not to my home necessarily, although it does seem familiar and comfortable, but to humanity's home. I have a chemical reaction to the earth and landscape; it is the place we were born and grew up as a species.

* * *

Our human ancestors evolved the ability for endurance running around two million years ago.[1] In *Why We Run,* Bernd Heinrich describes a cave painting he saw on a research trip to Zimbabwe:

> Painted onto the wall under the overhang was a succession of small, sticklike human figures in clear running stride. All were clutching delicate bows, quivers, and arrows.... [T]hen I noticed something more, and it sent my mind reeling. It was the figure farthest to the right, the one leading the progression. It had its hands thrown up in the air in the universal runner's gesture of triumph at the end of a race. This involuntary gesture is reflexive for most runners who have fought hard, who have breathed the heat and smelled the fire, and then felt the exhilaration of triumph over adversity.

For Heinrich, this image served as a reminder "that the roots of our running, our competitiveness, and our striving for excellence go back very far and very deep." When we run in nature, we reach back and touch our ancestors.

The roots of running go down to the very bedrock of our humanity. To run, we needed to walk, and to walk, we needed to walk on two legs — to become bipedal. Why and how did this happen? African apes live in trees. They are strong but slow. They have large hands, large feet, short arms — features that are important for climbing trees but are impediments to running.[2] They are quadrupeds, living and feeding on the forest floor.

You may have seen a chimpanzee knuckle walk, resting its forelimbs on flexed hands as it moves around on all four limbs. Knuckle walking allows primates to move as quadrupeds while still being well adapted to tree climbing. However, the strongly flexing hands of chimpanzees and gorillas are not able to match the extremely precise movements of our own very dexterous fingers.[3] Knuckle walking only allows for very slow movement; it does not make chimpanzees more agile on land. Knuckle walking wastes energy. It was an evolutionary strategy that led nowhere.

To become great runners, humans first had to become bipedal. This transition began with the last common ancestor (LCA) of humans and chimpanzees. Whether or not this ancestor was a knuckle walker is, for now, unknown. But one characteristic of this primate that is more certain is that it was built more for power than endurance. It is likely that its muscle groups were made up predominantly of fast-twitch fibres, which are well adapted for heavy lifting. It would have had more strength than *Homo sapiens* but less ability to cool itself, less energy efficiency, and limited ability to walk or run long distances.[4]

Fast-forward to four million years ago and the fossil record reveals my favourite human ancestors: the australopiths. In high school, I saw an image of a small, hairy primate chasing some kind of antelope progenitor with a spear, and I read the word *Australopithecus*. Saying it is like having ice in your mouth. The australopiths were a large group of early hominids who lived in Africa between one and four million years ago. They were the first of our ancestors to descend from the trees and begin life on just two legs.[5]

One million years later, a corner of East Africa echoed with the soft footfall of Lucy, an *Australopithecus afarensis* discovered in Ethiopia. She was a young but mature female and would have stood only three feet tall and weighed sixty pounds.[6] She shows features of the transition to bipedalism. I have looked in awe at reconstructions of her skull, which is so small and different from our own but is at the same time so human.

Lucy is a wonder. Unlike her ancestors' bodies, which were built to move on all fours, Lucy's knees and hips were better adapted for upright walking, and she had a more developed gluteus maximus muscle — a feature that helps prevent bipeds from tipping forward with each foot strike.[7] The large gluteus maximus is very active during running and has a small role in walking. The modern human body is unique in having hips that are slightly larger than the waist; this has resulted in part from running adaptations. The narrow waist also promotes a stable posture during running.

But Lucy did not have the figure of a modern woman. Her legs were short in comparison to her torso and arms — a feature that would have been an advantage for tree climbing. She was a woman of two worlds — the past and the future, the land and the trees. As Lucy and her descendants moved toward full bipedalism, they became progressively worse tree climbers. Modern humans are the only primate that is poorly suited to life high in the trees.[8] Although Lucy was much better suited to life in the trees than modern humans are, the fact that she was less well-adapted to that life may have been the cause of her death. After meticulously CT scanning her bone fragments, researchers proposed that she had been killed after falling from a tree. Lucy was a victim of her own pioneering transition from the trees to the land, not quite at home in either world.

Another discovery that unlocked more of the secrets of our blossoming bipedalism was made near Olduvai Gorge. Approximately 3.6 million years ago, a group of hominids, probably *Australopithecus afarensis*, walked across a layer of wet, cement-like volcanic ash that later hardened into fossil evidence.[9] These tracks are unequivocal evidence of bipedal primates trekking toward the Olduvai basin. An eighty-foot-long track of double prints is a testament to a couple marching in search of food or water or their companions.[10] We can learn from those footprints information about how weight was transmitted through the feet of that couple who lived so long ago. The feet seem to have been structured like ours, with similar arches and a similar big toe in lines with the others. But there are things that we will likely never know about the people who made those prints. Richard Dawkins, in *The Ancestor's Tale: A Pilgrimage to the Dawn of Evolution*, asks in reference to these footprints, "Who does not wonder what these individuals were to each other, whether they held hands or even talked, and what forgotten errand they shared in a Pliocene dawn?"

We were marching toward a human form built to stand, walk, and run upright on two feet. But why become bipedal? Bipedalism is precarious — once you start thinking about how unlikely it is, you wonder how it works at all. Stand up for a moment and think about how hard it is to stay upright. Do you feel dizzy? Now think about how difficult it would have been for our ancestors to run while being chased by sabre-toothed tigers or raiders from the next tribe. Why did they do it? Wouldn't it have been safer to get down on all fours and really move? Maybe, but that wasn't the path of human evolution.

Perhaps we became bipedal to carry more food on foraging trips; perhaps walking erect allowed us to move in shallow water or stand tall in savannah grass; or it kept us cooler when we stood upright in the sun, directly exposing only a fraction of our body to heat at a time when we had no technology to cool ourselves.[11] Being bipedal may have led to our becoming relatively hairless, as we needed hair only on our heads and shoulders to be protected from the sun when standing.

Charles Darwin thought we became bipedal so that we might carry tools to hunt and defend ourselves. What Darwin didn't know is that tools don't appear in the fossil record until about two million years after australopiths became bipedal, thus suggesting something else entirely drove this evolutionary change.[12] In light of this evidence, Darwin might agree with current ideas that a superior ability to hunt and gather while upright was probably the key driver.

Walking upright made early humans better hunter-gatherers, as they could travel much greater distances in search of sustenance. A big-city marathon runner can traverse a lot of ground and see all the big sites when running at a good pace for three hours. During humanity's transition to walking and running, the environment was changing, and this further drove evolution. Initially, Africa was warmer and wetter than it is today. During the Pliocene epoch, from 5.3 to 2.6 million years ago, Africa became cooler and drier, which thinned out the rainforests and promoted the growth of open woodlands and bushlands.

While many primates chose to stay in the relative safety of the deep forest, our ancestors ventured out of this comfortable niche, thus taking an enormous risk. New types of food had to be found while confronting the constant threat of new predators. Like children today, they preferred to eat fruit, but in this new environment they were forced to eat other types of plants as well. Foraging for such plants may have required more travel in open landscapes. So individuals better able to walk long distances and also climb whatever fruit-bearing trees remained would have fared better and, thus, been more likely to reproduce.[13]

It is a testament to the tenacity of our early ancestors that they were able to survive in this new landscape. But the fossil record is filled with the remains of those who did not survive. Indeed, one australopith skull fragment found in South Africa was punctured by a leopard's teeth, the body having been dragged across the ground.[14] A region of Ethiopia called Dikika has yielded further Paleolithic treasures including the tragic sight of a crouched skeleton of a three-year-old female *Australopithecus afarensis* who has been called Selam. Her skeleton is so well preserved that it seems she was washed away from her family by flood waters and buried immediately in soft mud.[15] CT scans of her inner ear show us that her semicircular canals are similar to those of apes and other australopiths, which indicates that while she was an upright walker, she did not have all the adaptations needed for fast running. Specialized developments in the inner ear, which helps to control balance, allow modern humans to keep our heads fairly stable while running.[16]

In 1984 another ancient tragedy was discovered — this one in the north of Kenya, at Lake Turkana, which also runs into the Ethiopian border. Excavators found the most complete skeleton of an early human ever discovered. The remains, which date back to approximately 1.5 million years ago, were identified as belonging to a *Homo erectus* boy thought to be around eight years old. Although young, he already stood five feet, three inches tall. He was lying face down in swampy mud.[17] He is known as the Nariokotome Boy. Unlike Lucy and Selam, he was better adapted to life on the ground. His narrow pelvis and longer limbs suggest he was more fully bipedal than earlier primates.[18] Preserved footprints from 1.5 million years ago found around the same lake reveal large hominid feet with a long stride and very modern foot anatomy.[19]

Changes to our feet, legs, and joints have been key to our ability to run. The plantar arch in the foot acts as a spring that returns energy generated during the weight-loading phase of our running stride.[20] The Achilles tendon and iliotibial band also serve as springs; they are tiny or absent on other primates but grew larger in our ancestors.[21] Our feet and toes became smaller as our legs became longer, and we evolved larger weight-bearing joints that could endure long runs without incurring damage.[22]

Two million years ago our ancestors evolved into *Homo erectus,* upright man, the first hunter-gatherers. In them, we can begin to glimpse figures more like ourselves. They lived in ever growing social conglomerations and used ever more complex technologies. It was they who first used fire to cook food and who first made tools, such as stone axes; they lived in bands and cared for the sick. They spread from Africa across Asia as far as China and Indonesia. They had larger brains, smaller teeth, longer legs, shorter arms, and modern feet.[23] They could run.

This changed everything. But in order to run for prolonged periods, the bodies of our ancestors had to prevent overheating. Four features contributed to this ability: the ability to sweat, an external nose, a way to cool the brain, and a thin and upright body.[24]

Consider our ability to sweat. Something few people realize is that all mammals, other than humans, use panting as their central strategy to dissipate heat. This strategy is not very effective, as the mouth and tongue provide only a small surface to dissipate heat.[25] Humans sweat from our entire skin surface — we can produce a lot of sweat. As we evolved, we lost most of our body hair and at the same time developed a very high number and density of sweat glands.[26] Sweating cools us because it takes a significant amount of energy to evaporate the sweat that develops on the skin surface.[27] We can sweat up to three litres an hour, and in a three-hour hunt or marathon, a fit person can lose up to 10 percent of their body weight through sweating without much risk of keeling over.[28]

Sometimes marathon kit bags include sponges that runners can dip into buckets of water and squeeze over themselves as they run. This water produces a momentary feeling of coolness, but it actually blocks the sweat glands and does not contribute to cooling at all. Being covered in water is a bit like being covered in hair, and evolution has selected for individuals with less hair. Think of how much of your body is exposed to the sun when you stand upright, particularly when the sun is high in the sky. Most of it hits your head and shoulders. Only 7 percent of the human body is exposed to direct sunlight when the body is upright, whereas a quadruped feels the sun on a much greater proportion of its body. With the loss of all that hair, sweat can be much more efficiently evaporated. This is critical if you are doing a lot of running and walking. Being without hair also helps to protect humans against parasites, such as lice, that hide in hair-covered places.[29]

Why did we need these adaptations to cool ourselves? Perhaps we evolved to forage in the heat specifically in order to avoid predators. Biologists paint a picture of early hominids walking long distances in the open while constantly being on the lookout for lions and sabretooth tigers. Like the cavemen of Arthur C. Clarke's *2001: A Space Odyssey*, their lives were marked by constant fear and real mortal threats. Thus, if early pre-humans could venture out in the hottest part of the day with their sun-exposed 7 percent body area conveniently covered in hair while the rest of their body sweated profusely, they could stay cool enough to forage while the big predators were resting in the shade.[30]

Even modern humans excel at sustained activity in the heat. Humans are the only species that can run a marathon on a day as hot as 30°C. Not even a horse or dog can match this feat, and it is unlikely that any prehistoric predator could either.[31] Most other mammals are good at sprinting but not as good at endurance activities. It defies belief, but we are even better at long-distance running than horses, particularly when the weather is hot. We evolved from animals with low metabolic capacity and rapidly improved both our metabolism and our ability to take up and use oxygen, a measure known as VO_2 max, which I explore later in the book.[32]

To survive in a hostile world, we developed the ability to sweat and to cool the air entering our bodies. We have a unique nose that brings air in at nearly a 90-degree angle relative to the nasal passages. This shape makes the air turbulent and cools it down as it enters the lungs. The lining of our respiratory system cools the air and adds moisture to bring it to a temperature of 37°C and a perfect level of humidity as it reaches the lungs.[33]

These adaptations were useful for foraging on hot days, but what about hunting? We were not vegetarian. I recently saw a poster at a country fair that showed a modern hunter holding a powerful rifle. The poster caption read "I didn't get to the top of the food chain to become a vegetarian." What is remarkable is that we were killing animals with only stones or sharpened sticks. We invented stone points five hundred thousand years ago and the bow and arrow one hundred thousand years ago. With only these weapons, hunters would have had to get very close to their prey, some of which were very dangerous, in order to kill them.

The theory here is that we basically ran the poor creatures to death through a practice called persistence hunting. Early humans would frighten their prey, perhaps wound them, and then keep following them until the animal overheated and collapsed. The hunters chasing these animals sweated and used their well-adapted noses to stay cool and their well-adapted bodies to keep running. Persistence hunting still occurs today; its use has been documented among hunter-gatherers in the Kalahari Desert. As the theory predicts, this hunting is done during the hottest part of the day.[34]

One amazing feature of modern humans is our ability to adapt to a variety of conditions. I believe a big reason for our success as a species is our multitude of talents, particularly our use of intelligence to take advantage of our upright posture and our agile hands to find and acquire food from an infinite variety of sources. We can run for long distances in the heat, but we can also swim in deep water. We can dig and carry, and we can throw with lethal power and accuracy.[35] More recently, our use of tools and more complex technology has allowed us to continue to differentiate ourselves from other species. In order for us to develop tools, we have needed to develop our brain capacity and cognitive abilities.

But the brain was slow to develop. Lucy could walk upright, but her brain was barely larger than that of a chimpanzee. The brain of *Homo erectus* was only slightly bigger, but it showed pivotal changes, such as an expansion of the part of the brain responsible for language.

A study comparing brain size and exercise capacity in a variety of mammals found that bigger brains are correlated with better exercise capacity. Thus, the superior ability of humans to undertake endurance activities may be linked to our superior cognitive abilities.[36]

This remarkable finding can be explained by considering the attributes that would have allowed ancient hunters to survive and thrive. They needed to be fit, to have endurance, but they also needed to be able to visualize the landscape and remember the locations of food sources and watering holes. Those with superior fitness and cognitive abilities were more successful at bringing home nutrients. The hunter-gatherers able to bring home more food would have had more mating opportunities — a classic example of sexual selection. More mating opportunities ensured the preservation and propagation of these traits.[37]

The brain is the most energy-hungry organ in the human body, consuming about a fifth of the body's caloric intake. As human brains enlarged, our caloric needs increased. Not only are our brains bigger than those of our ancient ancestors, but our bodies are also larger as well. Both of these developments have increased our need for nutrients.

Our skulls also had to change to make room for these growing brains. The large jaw muscles that enable the powerful bites of other primates also constrain the growth of the skull since they exert a strong force at their insertion points. In humans, a single mutation may have led to the weakening of the jaw muscles, which allowed our brains to grow. As we started to use tools to butcher animals, ate more nutritious food, and, much later, began to cook our food, a powerful bite became less important for survival.

The oldest evidence of hominids using fire to cook food stretches back only 450 thousand years. Fire made food better. Cooked food is easier to eat and easier to digest. Less time and effort are needed to eat it, and a smaller gut can be used to digest it. Cooking food allowed humans to more easily acquire the nutrients needed for brain development, and it also gave them more time to use these higher cognitive functions.[38]

A protein called brain-derived neurotrophic factor (BDNF) may have driven some of these changes. Much of the brain growth that took place over the course of human evolution occurred in the neocortex, the area that gives rise to language and allows for the development of culture through the production of symbols. BDNF may promote growth of the hippocampus and prefrontal cortex. These are areas of the brain involved in spatial mapping, decision-making, and the control of emotions such as fear and impulses to violence. BDNF is promoted by exercise and may be a reason physical activity is linked to improved cognitive function and reduced psychiatric illness, links we will explore in the coming chapters.[39]

Larger brains, possibly directed by BDNF, became capable of language, and language led to culture. In *Consilience: The Unity of Knowledge*, E.O. Wilson says these changes resulted in our "capacity to take possession of the planet." He traces the evolution of culture from the development of humans' ability to utilize fire 450 thousand years ago, to the ability to produce well-made tools 250 thousand years ago, to the invention of elaborate spearheads and daggers one hundred thousand years later, to the creation of breathtaking cave paintings and artifacts of ritual around thirty thousand years ago. For much of prehistory, our ancestors' bodies evolved faster than did their simple stone axes. Modern *Homo sapiens* evolved between two hundred thousand and one hundred thousand years ago. Ten thousand years ago, we developed agriculture. Since then, cultural evolution has accelerated at an exponential rate, and every year it seems to change faster and faster.

We almost did not survive as a species. Around seventy thousand years ago, the last Ice Age cooled the planet dramatically, and all our adaptations to dissipate heat, in particular our lack of fur, were suddenly big liabilities. In this new environment, our ancestors began to die out, likely due to starvation and exposure. By the end of the Ice Age, only ten thousand people remained on the entire planet — the population of a small town today. But these humans had fire, basic tools, and modern brains. The survivors clung to life and began to spread rapidly from East Africa. In the new and difficult environments they encountered, their incredible metabolism, resourcefulness, and adaptability came to the fore.

The first group followed the coast and crossed from modern-day Djibouti to Yemen then on to the coast of India and Southeast Asia. From there, small groups set sail, over time establishing new settlements on the archipelagos and islands of the western Pacific Ocean until some reached Australia, approximately fifty thousand years ago. Around that time, a second group left East Africa and headed to the Middle East and

Central Asia. From these areas, they moved into Europe and East Asia. Finally, during a time of great cold, following a frozen land bridge connecting Russia with Alaska, a group of Asian hunters crossed over into North America. They made their way south and had occupied the entire hemisphere by around ten thousand years ago.[40]

Life for these colonists, constantly making their way to new lands and encountering new threats while seeking new food sources, was unimaginably harsh. Those who were more settled also faced the vagaries of extreme weather conditions, persistent food scarcity, danger from predators, and threats from other humans. The physical demands on their bodies were constant. Imagine a day in the life of a Paleolithic human: each day they had to walk and run to gather food; visit or migrate to other campsites; carry children, animals, or their belongings; butcher meat; dig roots; erect shelters; collect firewood; shell nuts; and make tools. With what energy they had left over, they still managed to engage in social activities such as competitions, playing, dancing, wooing, and mating.

Just like modern humans, they would have experienced pleasure from neurochemicals released from this physical exertion, but they would have also suffered profound hunger and fatigue. Their physical activity alone burned through about 1,250 calories per day.[41] But their overall caloric needs were much higher. Male hunter-gatherers expended about 2,500 calories per day; females generally needed less, but when they were pregnant or lactating, would have needed up to one thousand calories more every day. In a time before birth control, women would have spent much of their lives pregnant or lactating. Acquiring this many calories was challenging, particularly for mothers who could gather about two thousand calories per day but relied on partners and family members for the additional calories they needed both for themselves and their young children. People lived very close to energy balance, and most would have suffered times of extreme hunger and nutritional deficiency.[42]

In her article "Physical Inactivity from the Viewpoint of Evolutionary Medicine," Sylvia Kirchengast describes the situation of our Paleolithic ancestors:

> For our ancestors, the motivating factors for a physically active lifestyle were not a desire for activity; the motivations were hunger and thirst. Physical activity was a major part of their lives because it was essential for surviving. Only physically active individuals were able to survive long enough to reproduce successfully and bring up their offspring to reproductive age.[43]

Paleolithic humans were more active than modern humans, and they were active in different ways. Rather than doing one thing over and over again, they did a range of activities similar to vigorous cross-training. They combined strength-based activities, such as carrying and chopping, with the aerobic activities of hunting and gathering. From what we've learned of the lifestyles of modern hunter-gatherers, men would hunt two to four non-consecutive days in a week, while women would gather for two to three days a week. This pattern has been called the "Paleolithic work rhythm."[44]

Everything changed again ten thousand years ago after the advent of agriculture, which marked the end of the Paleolithic period. The rise of agriculture during the Neolithic transition broke a pattern of activity that had been in place for roughly eighty-four thousand generations. Suddenly, energy acquisition and energy expenditure were no longer inextricably linked.[45] As humans learned to domesticate plants and animals, we were able to produce and even store surplus food. Most people gave up their nomadic lifestyles and lived in growing population centres, first in the Fertile Crescent, then across the globe. The great variety of the Paleolithic diet was replaced by carbohydrate-rich plants, such as rice, barley, and wheat.[46]

This transition was difficult. Neolithic skeletal remains show protein deficiency. People got shorter, due, at least in part, to malnutrition. New infectious diseases jumped the species barrier from recently domesticated animals.[47] We adapted slowly to this new way of life, but eventually most humans settled into a life based on farming and tending to animals. This pattern of activity and consumption remained relatively unchanged until the beginning of the Industrial Revolution, when physical activity became almost completely decoupled from food production and economic productivity.[48]

Every decade since the Industrial Revolution has seen the invention of new labour-saving devices and, with their adoption, a further decline in our physical activity. For most people today, little or no physical labour is required to acquire food. While our ancestors expended thousands of calories in order to get the nutrition they needed, modern humans expend virtually no calories. Whereas Paleolithic people burned 1,250 calories every day undertaking the activities of survival, people in industrialized regions today burn about 550 calories. At a time of great abundance of nutrients, we burn less than half as many calories through activity.[49] Cars, electric appliances, and the supermarket have made our lives more and more sweat-free. Just as our bodies were transformed by environmental changes in the Paleolithic period, so they are changing again today.

Between 1863 and 1970, American men of the same age and height gained 8.7 kilograms. Obesity rates more than doubled between 1970 and 2000 in the United States. Performing the same physical fitness tests, soldiers in the U.S. Army today cannot match the scores attained by their predecessors in 1946, and Westerners, in general, are physically weaker than our ancestors.[50] The superabundance of calorie-rich fast food sweetened with high-fructose corn syrup, combined with declining physical activity, are the obvious culprits.

Patterns of low physical activity start in childhood. Children are driven to school, sit in classrooms, watch too much TV, and do too little sport. Some European countries, like Holland and Denmark, promote active transport and plenty of outdoor play, but they are unusual.[51] My son was startled on a trip to Holland to see entire classes of young children panting and laughing as they followed their teachers on bikes along cycle paths and roads to their field trips. The sight is unimaginable in North America, where cars rule all roads and children are trapped by safety, speed, and comfort. Already in 1793, the German scholar Johann GutsMuths wrote that "[a]lmost all day is spent sitting still; how can young people's energy be developed?"[52] He developed concepts of natural education, training, and outdoor play, urging that we should let children "come out into the fresh air." More than two centuries later, we are beginning to hear the message.

The evidence that we are insufficiently active in the West, and increasingly across the globe, is clear. The average American takes five thousand steps per day, compared to 18,500 for an average Amish man living without modern technologies.[53] One third of the world's population — over two billion people — does not engage in sufficient exercise, defined as approximately 150 minutes per week of moderately intense activity for adults. One survey in 2008 found that 56 percent of Americans do no aerobic activity.[54]

Children need even more exercise, around one hour per day of moderate to vigorous activity. About two-thirds of American high school students do not meet minimum activity requirements.[55] Activity early in life can change the developmental trajectory of a child's body and mind. Their physical fitness as measured by VO_2 max is determined in part by childhood activity, as is peak bone strength and muscle mass. Exercise also makes children smarter, or, at the very least, better able to focus; those who are more active do better at school.[56]

The evidence that inactivity in children and adults is having negative consequences is also immense and growing. The Greek physician Hippocrates wrote 2,400 years ago: "That which is used, develops, and that which is not used, wastes away.... If there is any deficiency in food or exercise the body will fall sick."[57] Contemporary experts are sounding the alarm using a variety of colourful terms. The essence of their concern is that physical inactivity is the greatest threat to health in the twenty-first century. Karim Khan, a sports and exercise medicine researcher, has argued that low fitness may be responsible for more deaths than "smokadiabesity" — that is, smoking, diabetes, and obesity combined.[58]

Physical inactivity makes a person much more likely to have coronary heart disease, which can result in angina and heart attacks. Diabetes risk is greatly increased. It increases blood pressure, lowers healthy cholesterol, and increases the risk of stroke. The risks of colon and breast cancer are significantly raised among the inactive. Obesity, which mediates many other diseases, is strongly associated with low activity. In the elderly, low activity is associated with frailty, falls, reduced functional status, worsening mood, and increased dementia. Anxiety and depression are linked to low activity. Overall, physical inactivity makes us more likely to die at an earlier age and is thought to cause about 13 percent of premature deaths in the United States.[59] Globally, inactivity is thought to cause 9 percent of premature deaths, or around fifty-seven million deaths in 2008.

The science journalist Gretchen Reynolds summarizes the situation by pointing out that as science continues to amass evidence for the benefits of activity, citizens of industrialized countries have become "the most sedentary groups of humans ever to exist."[60] And even among people who are active for part of the day, sitting, what you may be doing right now, can be harmful. Adults in industrialized regions spend between 55 percent and 70 percent of their day sedentary, which is about nine to eleven hours of sitting.[61] More sitting is worse. Adults sitting more than ten hours a day have a 34 percent higher mortality risk, even after taking physical activity into account. Overall, sitting contributes to about 6 percent of all deaths.[62]

Even worse than sitting is prolonged bed rest, such as when a person is hospitalized, which provides us with evidence of the harms of extreme inactivity. The body responds very badly to this situation. Within a few hours, pooling blood can clot, leading to deep vein thrombosis and pulmonary embolism, a potentially fatal condition. Within a few days, insulin sensitivity plummets throughout the body. People become constipated — as my patients learn when they increase their activity and tell me that their chronic constipation problems have miraculously resolved. Within a few weeks, heart function declines, as evidenced by worsening stroke volume, cardiac output, and VO_2 max. Bones lose mass at ten times their normal rate. Skeletal muscles atrophy. The body hates inactivity.[63]

And yet, the evolutionary biologist Daniel Lieberman thinks we may have evolved to be physically inactive. As I will explore in later chapters, rest is an essential part of remaining healthy. So, while we were selected by evolution to be become bipedal and develop incredible endurance, we were also adapted to rest. While hunter-gatherers spent a lot of time looking for food and attending to the stuff of survival, they also spent time sitting, resting, eating, and napping.[64] When you live very close to the energy balance, any wasteful use of energy can make the difference between starvation and survival. And just like communities that rely on solar or wind power are learning to store energy in massive batteries to smooth out energy delivery, so our bodies adapted to store as much fat as possible as insurance against tough times. Females evolved to do this particularly well since high amounts of energy are needed for reproduction and child care. Female hunter-gatherers have 15–25 percent body fat, compared to 10–15 percent in men and only 5–8 percent body fat in other primates.[65]

Lieberman points out that there was never any selective pressure to avoid physical inactivity or obesity because we didn't evolve in a world where prolonged inactivity was an option. In fact, there was strong selection for us to have more fat compared with other mammals.[66]

Early humans evolved to walk and run; later, their brains grew larger, more complex, turning into something akin to a twenty-five-watt computer. With that advanced brain, humans have been able to develop tools, technology, and culture, all of which have enabled our incredible success in spreading across the globe. For 99 percent of our evolutionary history, humans were hunter-gatherers. We lived in small bands and stored any small energy surplus we could find as body fat. Culture and technology allowed us to change the world to such an extent that the acquisition of energy was no longer linked to the expenditure of energy. We have increased the amount we eat while expending less energy to acquire food. This imbalance has changed our bodies, resulting in obesity and chronic diseases. Unless we can change our genes, our brain, or our metabolism, we need to rediscover the joys of an active life to mitigate the harmful effects of the world we have created.

With a knowledge of how our bodies move, it is possible to discover how exercise, like endurance running, can allow us to marry the products of human ingenuity with peak physical well-being.

II RUNNING INTO MEDICINE AND SCIENCE

I ran through childhood, and when I was eleven, I entered my first organized race. It was a "biathlon" that began with a swim in the Indian Ocean and finished with a 5K run. One hot Sunday morning, many of the expatriates living in Dar es Salaam gathered at the start line. Next to me was Gavin, a classmate from the international school in the centre of the dusty city. The race began and I ran down the ramp into the sea. As I swam through the swells, gasping for air, my fear evoked in my mind images of capsized ships and underwater creatures. I thought about the small boat with four crew that had recently sunk on the journey from Zanzibar back to the mainland. I thought about the decrepit hydrofoil I had travelled on to cross the thirty-six-kilometre channel to the exotic island. I pushed through the water, feeling the swells urging me sideways even as I kicked forward. I thought of our last visit to Zanzibar, sitting in the hotel lobby while outside I could hear waves and smell musty cloves in the night air.

We emerged from the ocean, ran up the boat ramp of the local yacht club, and changed into our running shoes under the intense morning sun. The Tanzania of my childhood was a hot and humid land. At night the lightning of summer storms split the sky. I watched from my bedroom window, hearing the thunder and the hot rain banging against the slatted windowpanes. The sky was immense, and the streaks of electricity reached down to the flat dirt of the city. Years later I would think of those nights when I read a description in J.M. Coetzee's memoir, *Boyhood*: "What he would write if he could … would be something darker, something that, once it began to flow from his pen, would spread across the page out of control, like spilt ink. Like spilt ink, like shadows racing across the face of still water, like lightning crackling across the sky."

We ran through the hot morning along dusty unpaved streets. I felt the sun pushing me into the ground. My legs were heavy. I willed myself on, running alongside Gavin. We were moving together until, steps from the finish line, he caught his foot and fell. There was blood on his right knee. I stopped and together we walked the rest of the way. He was in pain, but we were both elated to finish. We ate oranges and boiled eggs. I saw in Gavin's eyes the exhilaration of the race, even as the blood oozed from his leg.

I kept running, and when I was thirteen, we moved to Egypt. One winter my family and I drove from Cairo to the Sinai Peninsula, the scrap of land at the top of the Red Sea bridging Africa to the Middle East. We stayed at a small hostel at the base of Mount Sinai. The practice of those staying in the hostel was to awake several hours before dawn and hike to the summit to witness sunrise over the desert. Although groggy with sleep, my brothers and I raced up the mountain. We were exhilarated by the sharp smell of eucalyptus and the cold, dry desert air. I think of the writer Peter Matthiessen who, in *The Snow Leopard*, a memoir of his own desert journey fifty years earlier, described the cold of the desert as "the cold of the dark universe descended."

We reached the summit well before sunrise and were hit by the cold. The constellations above us were clearly visible, much more distinct than from our neighbourhood in the shining metropolis of Cairo. A man in a small, makeshift hut just large enough for one person sold hot chocolate, which we gratefully accepted in an attempt to warm ourselves. Our parents joined us at the summit, and in the company of dozens of others, we witnessed the sun begin to light up the horizon as the Earth spun into another day in the Middle East.

I joined the cross-country team at my school in Cairo in the ninth grade. I fell in with a group of three American boys — Tyler, Mikey, and Jonah. This was a coup because Tyler and Jonah were the fastest boys on the team. They spoke knowingly about the importance of carbohydrates, and their success in races bore out their cool assurance. When I started training with them, I could hardly run. I could sprint for a few breathless seconds and I loved to play outside in the two fields surrounded by our school's running track, but I wasn't a runner.

There is a photo of me in the school yearbook from grade eight that reveals my humble beginnings. I had decided to run a 5K race in the desert. Looking back, I realize that the run itself was not what inspired me to participate in the event; it was the location of the run — it was held in the Petrified Forest — that drew me in. This natural formation was strewn endlessly with what appeared to be rocks but were, on closer inspection, great fistfuls of petrified wood. The race was painful, as I didn't know how to find my rhythm. I gasped for air and felt my body slow as I approached the end. The yearbook photo shows me with red cheeks, a pained look on my face, with the caption, "Brodie struggles to finish the race." I had a long way to go.

The next year, on the cross-country team, I began to find my legs. We trained on the school grounds and in the neighbourhood. The four of us gossiped and sang our way through our long runs. One afternoon I was leaving practice and felt buoyant, a new sensation I couldn't quite identify. "It's the runner's high," Tamara, one of my classmates and an incredible athlete herself, told me. It was an uplifting experience, and years later, I would come to understand the science underlying this natural euphoria.

The first cross-country race at the end of the season was held in the desert. Our competitors were dozens of boys from other schools in the city. We took buses out to a long narrow rift in the landscape. It was a cool, bright day, and the wind blew down the rift. I had been here before. One night, I had gone camping with my four best friends. We climbed the escarpment and found a cave. We crept inside until we realized the cave was full of hundreds of tiny bats and ran out yelling with feverish excitement.

When the race started, I was with Mikey. Tyler and Jonah ran ahead — they were leading the pack. My breathing was heavy, but I pushed through. The sand was firm underfoot. Running on the desert floor is the most incredible feeling. The surroundings blurred as I focused on the terrain immediately in front of me, on keeping up with Mikey, on the competitors. My legs hurt; my insides hurt; it was hard to keep moving. We ran out 2,500 metres then back. Afterward, we drank water and caught our breath. We did well, but there would be another race the next day on a grass running track in the centre of the city.

The next day, we arrived at an old colonial sports facility. The track was four hundred metres and we would do twelve laps, just short of five kilometres. This time, I believed I could win. The dry grass crunched audibly underfoot in the Egyptian winter. This time I was with the front of the pack throughout the race. I felt fast, nothing hurt, and I pictured myself running as if I were watching from above. I saw myself on the track flanked by six boys all pushing toward the end. I didn't win, but I finished with my fastest time yet and felt victorious.

The week after our cross-country meet, we were running the mile in gym class. I had always been an average miler, but cross-country had changed that. This time I started at the front of the class and maintained the lead. Mazed, an Egyptian classmate who had always been the king of running in gym class, kept up with me for the first half. As we reached the final lap of the track, he began to sprint. I matched his pace and then exceeded it. My arms pumped; my breath was coming fast. I felt the speed. I beat him with one hundred metres to spare. My gym teacher came over to congratulate me. "That was fast," he gasped. In fact, it was probably the fastest I'd ever be, as two weeks later, cross-country season was over, and I wouldn't run regularly again for another fifteen years.

Why did I stop running? I wanted to run in soccer, in tennis, and in baseball, but not more. Some evenings after school I'd come back to the track and run laps. I did this more out of habit from cross-country than for enjoyment. So many other things interested me. I revelled in theatre and spent much of my free time rehearsing and learning lines. Running wasn't part of my identity. It wasn't enough for me at that moment in my life.

We moved to Wales when I was entering grade eleven, a challenging time to start at a new school in a new country. I cycled around the countryside on my own. I walked and hiked the hills and along the coastal paths. After the rich social scene of my school in Cairo, my comprehensive school in the small Welsh town of Lampeter was lonely. I spent much of my time reading. We then moved back to Canada, and I continued to cycle. Running never occurred to me. I started university in Vancouver, but I hardly exercised beyond simple walking or cycling to go downtown or to a nearby cafe. I was so absorbed in my academics; I spent every minute studying, reading, and writing for the school newspaper. I moved to Montreal and finished my undergraduate degree at McGill. I decided to study science and taught chemistry for the medical entrance exam.

I met Melissa, who ran around Montreal's Laurier Park next to her apartment on Brébeuf Street. She told me that once she found her rhythm, she felt she could run forever. For the first five years of our relationship, she was the runner. We moved to the United Kingdom and studied for a year at Cambridge. We had our own flat on the second floor of a row of houses at 56 Eltisley Avenue. Ted Hughes and Sylvia Plath had lived right next door when they first lived together in Cambridge. Years later Melissa read me the poem "55 Eltisley Avenue" from Hughes's collection of letters to Sylvia.

From Eltisley, it was only a two-minute jog to a beautiful expanse of green space that follows the River Cam to the village of Grantchester. One Saturday afternoon, after hours bent over our desks reading academic papers, Melissa convinced me to go for a run. I hadn't been running in ten years. We headed out toward Grantchester, and I overheated immediately and gasped for air. I was wearing sweatpants and a sweatshirt, and only years later did I learn how much heat the body generates while running. I was hot, my stomach hurt, and I barely lasted fifteen minutes. I couldn't fathom why anyone would choose to run. We did not go running again. Instead, we cycled around the city and played tennis at the courts of nearby colleges. We explored the countryside and came to love the ancient and modern university as we brought home bags of groceries suspended from our handlebars.

Fourteen years after first setting foot in Cambridge, I returned one late October afternoon by train. I walked the crowded streets, checked in to a guest room at my old college, and immediately changed into my black running tights and a long-sleeved blue running shirt my wife's sisters had given me one Christmas. They had embroidered the words *You Can Do It* on the end of the right sleeve. I tied the laces on my mauve Nike running shoes and began running. Although older, I was now a runner. That afternoon and on into the evening I ran every corner of Cambridge I had neglected in my foolish youth. I ran past our old house on Eltisley Avenue, along the River Cam toward Grantchester, along the Backs past King's College and Trinity before heading into the centre of the town then along Market Street until, desperate for sustenance, I stopped in a bakery and devoured a sticky bun.

England has a rich history of running. The first official athletic records date from a race between Oxford and Cambridge in 1864. Of course, foot races had been held at fairs and tournaments for centuries before that, but the records of these are almost non-existent. The distances run and the times noted for them are completely unreliable. As industrialization spread, however, sport became increasingly quantified and technical, following such innovations as the standardization of distances and the use of reliable timekeepers. It was from this world of amateur gentlemen athletes that Roger Bannister emerged.

Like many runners of his day, Bannister wanted to break the four-minute mile record. He studied physiology intensively while undertaking his medical degree. He was fascinated by the science of endurance. He adjusted the speed and gradient of a treadmill, monitored his body temperature, blood acidity, and oxygen intake, and basically used his own body as a tool to learn about the limits of human performance. He was a popular presence in the university and became president of the Oxford University Athletics Club, a position that allowed him to direct the construction of a new running track at Iffley Road.

On the morning of May 6, 1954, Bannister went to the laboratory in the basement of his London training hospital. There he found a grindstone, on which he sharpened the spikes on his handmade running shoes. He covered the soles in graphite to prevent dirt from sticking to them. He took the train from London to Oxford and prepared to run at the Iffley Road track. There would be six men in the race. Two runners were his friends and pacers: Chris Chataway and Chris Brasher. It was a cool and blustery day, and it looked as though the conditions wouldn't favour a fast time.

The wind died down. The crowd was briefly silent as the sound of the starting gun echoed through the afternoon. Brasher led for the first two laps. He paced Bannister perfectly. Then Chataway took over. As they entered the final lap, the clock read 3:00.4. In the last half lap, Bannister unleashed his powerful stride. He pushed beyond the normal limits; his will was in direct control of his body. He pushed his chest through the tape. Immediately collapsing into the arms of another runner, he did not know what he had done. After a few agonizing minutes, the time was announced as a new "European, British Empire, and world's record." He had run the mile in 3 minutes, 59.4 seconds.

Forty-six days later, an Australian named John Landy ran a mile in 3 minutes, 57.9 seconds. In fact, once Bannister broke through the barrier, more runners followed in the years to come. But he was first, and that made all the difference. And indeed, Bannister earned his place in running lore because of what came next.

In August of that same year — 1954 — he raced John Landy at the Commonwealth Games in Vancouver. It was called the Race of the Century, and the buildup was followed around the world. One hundred million people listened to the race live as it was broadcast on the radio. The race was also filmed, and one afternoon recently, I watched the grainy footage while sitting in my garden. Landy took an early lead, and Bannister trailed him for much of the race. In the last ninety yards,

Landy looked to his left to check on Bannister's position, and at that very moment Bannister passed him on the right. The two men sprinted the final seconds to the finish line, with Landy unable to catch Bannister. Bannister finished in 3 minutes, 58.8 seconds; Landy came in at 3:59.6. It was the first time two runners had beaten four minutes in a race. It is exhilarating to watch even now, over sixty years later.

Following Bannister's path, Melissa and I decided to pursue medicine. We were both accepted to medical school at the University of Toronto, and we realized our lives would change. We moved to the heart of the city. It was our first time living in Toronto. We explored the neighbourhoods, visited the tiny parts of the Art Gallery of Ontario that were open while it was being reinvented by the architect Frank Gehry, and met the classmates who were to become our closest friends. We went to the medical school building to pick up our registration packages, and I had a nagging fear that our names would not be on the list. Fortunately, they were.

Medical school — like training for a marathon, like learning a new sport — changes a person. The four years I spent in the classrooms, clinics, and hospitals of Toronto were transformative. Because we would graduate in 2009, we were the class of "OT9," and those three characters became our identity.

For our very first lab, we dissected the mediastinum of a woman who had donated her body to medical science. It was humbling. I didn't even know what the mediastinum was before that time. I discovered it is the collection of the heart; the aorta, through which all oxygenated blood flows to the body; the *vena cava*, through which deoxygenated blood flows back to the heart; the esophagus; the trachea; a handful of nerves; and a scattering of lymph nodes. I didn't know there was so much inside the human chest. The next two months of medical school were consumed by anatomy and basic physiology. Many of my peers had studied some or all these subjects in detail before, but I was exploring facets of humanity I had never previously contemplated.

We began to ask questions that we had not considered before about how the body works. During our block on the gastrointestinal system, one of my classmates asked our anatomy teacher, "When does food moving through the intestines become stool?" This stumped our normally quick-witted instructor. When does food become stool? We agreed that this was likely a philosophical quandary and returned to our studies. Another day, while learning about the reproductive system, the same classmate asserted incredulously, "You mean women don't have prostates?" We had to think about this — do women have prostates? No, it seems, they do not.

Even more transformative was an introduction to a scientific way of thinking about medicine and, by extension, about the world. Reading about the history of medicine today leaves me ashamed of the magnitude of harm that physicians have inflicted on their patients for most of human history (while providing almost no benefit). The scientific revolution and the rise of Enlightenment values of reason and the questioning of accepted authority began to change the way medicine was practised. However, it was only in the twentieth century that the benefits offered by medical treatments finally began to outweigh the damages caused. This shift occurred as medicine embraced the fundamental tenets of science: to objectively understand and explain the world.

This drive has become embodied in the concept of "evidence-based medicine." In our lectures, we were taught to interpret and critique the scientific literature supporting certain explanations of disease or specific treatment recommendations. If a pharmaceutical company says its new medication reduces the risk of stroke, we have to ask first whether that is seen in the raw data from clinical trials, if any differences make biological sense, if they are statistically valid, and, finally, if they are clinically meaningful.

To understand something like the associations between physical inactivity and health, we have to be sure that one is causing the other, that they are not simply occurring at the same time. For example, you could argue that the development of the internet has come at the same time as rising obesity and diabetes rates, but that does not mean one caused the other. We were taught to question our own physical exam skills. For example, if you hear crackles or wheezes in a patient's lungs, how certain can you be of a diagnosis such as pneumonia or heart failure? In many cases, the answers are very humbling.

There is a concept in some environmental or anti-technology movements about the "arrogance" of science. What I learned in class and continuously see in the scientific literature is the profound humility of scientists who, like physicians, know that much of what was considered true in the past has been altered or upended by the emergence of new evidence. The fact that what was considered true in the past has been discovered to be incorrect, or to have only partial validity, does not mean we are in a postmodern sea completely devoid of objective truth. As I heard one scientist say, "Science put twelve men on the moon and brought them all home safely." There is an objective reality. However, we can always get a clearer picture of that reality; we can turn up the magnification on the microscope, look deeper and deeper into the closely guarded secrets of cells, bodies, and the universe at large.

Technological innovations have allowed doctors to offer better health care, and scientific advances have helped to solve problems such as cold, hunger, and disease; however, "progress" has also created new problems. As cars became faster and more affordable, the number of road accidents has increased. As a result of improved highway infrastructure and vehicle safety, we now burn too few calories through physical inactivity. This problem, in turn, has another solution, presumably some combination of increasing active transport exercise and reducing fat and sugar intake. My early classes in evidence-based medicine have given me a lens through which to view health and other social problems using science and evidence.

After we learned anatomy, we began a block entitled Metabolism and Nutrition. Our instructor had a hyperactive mind and delivered lectures like a machine gun spewing forth knowledge and spent shells. It was with him that I first learned about the physiology of running. To illustrate the production of energy at the cellular level, our instructor used the example of a sixty-kilogram woman planning to run a marathon. We calculated her energy needs and predicted when in the race she would transition from aerobic (utilizing oxygen) to anaerobic (without oxygen) metabolism. As

I listened to the lecture, I could imagine this theoretical woman running the marathon, her muscles consuming her body's glycogen (a form of glucose used by the body to store energy), devouring raw material like a hungry army; and as I considered how she sweated and mobilized her reserves, I saw inside the science of running for the first time.

Where does the spark of movement first occur? Is it in the mind — is it the will to run — or is it in the muscle with the contraction of muscle fibres? Gretchen Reynolds writes of her own discovery of running while at university:

> After a few months, I'd reach the fields, breathing easily now, and keep going, three, four, five times around the ploughed rectangles, and then still un-tired, run home. In the last few blocks, I'd sometimes stretch into a sprint. Without my telling them what to do, my knees would rise and my arms would pump. I'd toe off hard, feeling powerful and fast ... suddenly I had physical competence and even grace. My thighs bunched and lengthened with unselfconscious animal beauty. Who knew they could do that?[1]

After she decided to run, a shimmering cascade of factors and the messengers of neuromotor control oversaw the flow of calcium and the contraction of actin and myosin, which resulted in the bunching of those muscles.

Our skeletal muscle is central to our physical strength. Skeletal muscle is built of communities of thousands of cells. It stretches from tendon to tendon. Different fibres are faced with a range of tasks, from low-demand activities like walking and sitting upright to powerful blasts of high-amplitude work like jumping or heavy lifting.[2]

In our first year, we covered the physiology of respiration, cardiac output, circulation, and the mechanical action of the army of molecular machines that move our bodies. The body must adapt quickly and precisely to changes in the demand for oxygen, the production of acids, and the generation of heat. Our teachers showed us the equations for cardiac output, explaining that it is a function of heart rate and stroke volume. Cardiac output increases during exercise and is usually *the* limiting factor in determining a person's maximum oxygen uptake (VO_2 max). VO_2 max is often discussed in running circles and is considered the single best measure of cardiovascular fitness. VO_2 max is determined by genetics and childhood activity but can be improved with targeted training.

Stroke volume — the amount of blood one beat of the heart can push into the body — is the critical factor in determining VO_2 max. Athletes speak knowingly about their heart rates. A lower resting heart rate is a marker of aerobic fitness. This is because as a person exercises, their heart becomes bigger and stronger and thus increases its stroke volume. It can therefore push as much blood as the body needs by pumping at fifty to sixty beats per minute. On the other hand, a weaker heart will have to beat seventy to ninety beats per minute to do the same job.

The blood must travel through the lungs to pick up oxygen for delivery to the body. The cardiac output of a high-performance athlete can be nearly double the output of a less active person. Thus, with up to forty litres of blood pumping through an athlete's heart every minute, the red blood cells are travelling through the blood vessels in the lungs at lightning speed. It seems almost inconceivable that there would be time for the blood to pick up oxygen as they blast through the tiny pulmonary capillaries. But the transfer of oxygen across the alveoli (tiny air sacs) of the lungs is so beautifully orchestrated that, even with intense exertion, the body can keep the levels of oxygen and carbon dioxide in the blood at levels that are compatible with life.

The ability of the blood to carry oxygen also contributes to the final value of a person's VO_2 max. This is why athletes engage in blood doping — by removing, storing, then re-infusing red blood cells, they can artificially increase their ability to carry oxygen. In this way, cheaters can increase their VO_2 max by up to 9 percent.[3]

You can test your VO_2 max, but you should be prepared to suffer. While either running on a treadmill or riding an exercise bike, you need to work your way up your oxygen uptake curve through harder and faster exertion until you reach the point at which, although you are working harder, your oxygen uptake has plateaued because your body cannot do any better — that is your VO_2 max.

Your VO_2 max is measured in litres of oxygen absorbed per minute, which is divided by a person's weight (measured in kilograms) to recognize different levels for different size people. The average VO_2 max for a normal thirty-year-old man is around 36 L/min/kg and declines over time to around 30 by age sixty-five. In a woman, it declines from 30 to 22 L/min/kg over the same time.

Another important measure is lactate threshold. That is the level of oxygen uptake (VO_2) at which point lactate starts spilling into your muscles. Most elite athletes will compete just below their lactate threshold, which correlates with about 75 percent of the VO_2 max.

Our muscles are built from slow-twitch and fast-twitch fibres. Slow-twitch fibres can operate for long periods of time when the body is performing low-intensity endurance work. Fast-twitch fibres are used for short bursts of powerful movement. Different muscles in the body have different blends of slow- and fast-twitch fibres. Exercise can change the proportion of fibre types within a given muscle.

Exercise also has profound effects on the heart and circulatory system. Serious athletes have a bigger left ventricle, the part of the heart responsible for pumping blood throughout the body, and while these hearts may even look *too* large on X-rays, they function beautifully. The cardiac muscle fibres themselves become much larger and capable of much stronger contractions. The combined effect of strong muscle cells and a larger pump leads to increased stroke volume, thus allowing an athlete's heart to send huge amounts of blood to the muscles during intense activity.[4]

This transport of oxygenated blood is made more efficient in part because exercise induces the growth of new capillaries to the muscles. Exercise is the best treatment for blockage of arteries, called peripheral artery disease, as these new blood vessels grow to bypass blockages.

A vascular surgeon I was training with used the traffic analogy. As he told a sixty-three-year-old man with cold and painful legs as a result of peripheral blockages, "If there's too much traffic on one road, you build more lanes or other roads to bypass the traffic — that's what exercise does to your arteries."

One day an instructor was late for a physical exam session in the building across the street from the hospital. When he arrived, he was flushed and breathing hard. "I guess I'm out of shape," he said through shallow breaths.

Many of us have had the experience of struggling to breathe after a few flights of stairs only to find the same exertion considerably easier after a period of training. Our lungs become more efficient with exercise. They need to work less hard to move the same amount of oxygen or carbon dioxide. This leads to improvements in that key value, VO_2 max. Exercise allows us to use and distribute more oxygen to our entire body.[5]

Endurance training leads to the production of more and bigger mitochondria, the part of the cell that helps release energy from nutrients. Training expands the capillary bed supplying the muscles, increases the ability of skeletal muscle to store glycogen, and improves the ability of muscles to use fat as an energy source.[6]

Another mechanism that plays a role is *autophagy*, the process by which cells break down damaged parts of the cell. Exercise leads to a big rise in autophagy in skeletal muscle and other tissues. Mice that have been genetically modified to lack normal autophagy have much worse exercise capacity.[7] So, while exercise is stressful on the body, this stress encourages the body to clean up poorly functioning components, which in turn results in overall better function.

Another way exercise makes us stronger at the molecular level is by reducing oxidative stress, a type of inflammation that can result in cellular and DNA damage. When lab mice were mutated to lack the ability to control stress from oxidation, they went on to develop features of premature aging and died young. However, if they were allowed to exercise, there was nearly complete reversal of their aging features and they lived normal lives.

Paradoxically, exercise also reduces oxidative stress in cells since it induces the production of reactive oxygen species such as superoxide. The response to these dangerous oxidants is the stimulation of important antioxidant enzymes that protect cells from such damage. These enzymes remain at heightened levels long after exercise, giving the body extra protection against damage to protein and DNA. Endurance exercise leads to such protective responses in all major parts of our body's cells.[8]

A final and fascinating way in which exercise changes the body is through the secretory and signalling role of muscles. Only in the past twenty years have we realized that the muscles secrete signalling factors called *myokines* into the bloodstream. Muscle is the largest organ of the body and consumes up to 80 percent of cardiac output during peak exercise. Muscles allow animals to function and survive. When there is demand for more muscle, the muscle itself can cause cascades of changes through the body by releasing myokines, which attach to receptors on the liver, pancreas, bones, immune system, brain, and on the muscle itself.[9]

Some days of medical school felt like a marathon. Full days of lectures and labs were followed by hours in the library. For the first two years we spent almost every weekend in the library. In the final two years we began our clinical rotations, spending a month at a time as general surgery clerks or pediatric clerks or psychiatry clerks. I knew I wanted to work in primary care. I flirted with emergency medicine, but my main focus was global health and the health of the homeless. I had seen how my homeless patients suffered disproportionately from alcohol and opioid addiction, as well as HIV and other infectious diseases.

One day my supervisor asked me to meet him at a shelter on George Street, a few blocks from St. Michael's Hospital. Seaton House is the largest men's homeless shelter in Toronto. I walked from our apartment near the Eaton Centre, turned left on Dundas Street, and entered another world. Over my next few visits to the shelter, I realized that in the middle of Canada's richest city people suffered with pathologies that would not be out of place in a developing country or an earlier era. I diagnosed and treated patients with tuberculosis, trench foot, completely uncontrolled HIV, abscesses from injection drug use, and end-stage liver diseases. I still yearned to work in global health, but I learned that I did not have to set foot outside of urban Canada to find patients in need. The HIV and addiction doctors I worked with during those early years of training inspired me and set me on track to my current work.

As my understanding and experience of human health and disease grew, I repeatedly thought about how to be healthier myself. Even among my medical school classmates, we practised a huge range of what I learned to call "health behaviours." These behaviours included minimal exercise, terrible diets high in processed sugars and fat, and, in some cases, excessive alcohol consumption. Some things had changed — for example, none of my classmates were heavy smokers as far as I knew, a habit that would have been unremarkable one or two generations before. But we were definitely not paragons of good health.

When I moved to Ottawa for residency, I started cycling, but I felt a gnawing and persistent sense of underachievement. I would see people out for long runs on the canal path and feel awed by their courage — to be that far from home with only your legs to get you home seemed crazy. I had found that going to the gym, biking, walking, and hiking all made me feel good. I had runner's envy, but I still didn't believe I could go farther. The shadow of inactivity was looming over me — until one day I started running again.

The final push came from my brothers. My older brother, Alex, lived in Vancouver, and one day as we spoke on the phone, he told me he had started running and was training for a marathon. He ran a 10K race in Vancouver in a blistering thirty-nine minutes. He completed the marathon in less than four hours. He sent me a picture from the race. In the photo he was wearing shorts, sporting a medal, and looking happy. The picture made a big impact. Everything about it was incongruous. Growing up, Alex was extremely cerebral, gifted at music and foreign languages, and he was always reading. He would take me to second-hand bookshops and tell me about James Joyce and encourage me to read Kwame Nkrumah and Frantz Fanon. He performed a one-man show about Vincent van Gogh's life and played a Middle Eastern instrument called the *oud*. He certainly did not run or wear shorts. But in the picture he looked so happy.

Then my younger brother, Sascha, ran the Warsaw Marathon, and I began to feel left behind. I remembered my days running cross-country. Some nights, when I was too keyed up to relax, I decided to try to run along the river. From my house I turned into Windsor Park, followed a trail along the Rideau River, across Billings Bridge, then home. It took about half an hour and after a time it began to feel good. I listened to the same album by a Montreal singer called Ian Kelly over and over again. Sometimes I broke into a sprint, experimenting with this new way of being. Every time I ran, I knew I was slipping deeper into it, but I couldn't visualize how to go farther. I couldn't visualize it until it happened.

I was sitting at my desk at home talking to Sascha on Skype. He told me he was using a free running app on his phone that included training programs and tracked his progress. I listened intently; a light went on in my mind. He talked some more about his runs through the suburbs of Warsaw, and I realized that this was it. This was the key! I would use technology to take the final step toward becoming a runner. The ubiquitous screen, the computer we all carry with us, could actually make me run.

With mounting excitement, I downloaded the app and set my first goal — to run a 10K race in four months' time. The next day Melissa and I had planned to go away together for the weekend. Before we left, I slipped out of the house for my first programmed run. I felt scared, unsure what would happen on this first forty-minute run. Forty minutes seemed a long time. I ran slowly and carefully. I felt good. I could do this. According to my running app, that was the day I was born as a runner. That was the day it began to track my distance run, my calories burned, and the hours I spent on the road.

But all those wasted years! As I grew as a runner, I thought about what might have been if some other act of chance had set me on this track earlier. I had already seen the power of serendipity, as with my decision to go into the pre-medical sciences all those years ago. If I had been a runner back then, what else could I have accomplished? I was overcome with visions of running on the McGill cross-country team or running the rural roads of Cambridge, my lissome teammates at my side urgently pushing toward some never to be known victory. Oh, such regret! But it was not to be.

In his book about running, *What I Talk About When I Talk About Running*, the Japanese author Haruki Murakami describes his own birth as a runner at age thirty-three. He believes that age "may be a kind of crossroads in life." Alex and I both began running seriously in our early thirties. Sascha, being the youngest brother, has always been precocious — he started in his late twenties. But my day came in the end, and once I started, I did not look back, though it wasn't always easy from that day. After my first 10K race, I felt overwhelmed. I began to suffer from abdominal pain and cramping each time I trained. I thought maybe I wasn't cut out for running. Some days I walked home because I just couldn't keep going. It was strange, unnerving. I wasn't in total control of my body. But I willed it on, I pushed through, and soon running was, once again, a joy.

III RUNNING AND PHYSICAL HEALTH

Almost two thousand years ago, the ancient Greek physician Galen linked exercise and health. Galen directed a patient to lose weight "by making him run every morning until he fell into a profuse sweat."[1] But it was not through running alone that his patient improved. Galen further describes the treatment: "I then had him rubbed hard and put into a warm bath; after which I ordered him a small breakfast and sent him to the warm bath a second time. Some hours after, I permitted him to eat freely of food, which afforded but little nourishment; and lastly, set him to some work, which he was accustomed to for the remaining part of the day."[2]

Galen's method was idiosyncratic; his prescription of running likely had more beneficial impact than all those warm baths and the hard rub.

Using molecular and genetic tools, modern science reveals that exercise releases myokines and other elements that transmute activity into better health and stronger bodies.[3] Few of my patients believe me when I tell them that if we could distill the health benefits of exercise into a pill, it would be the most powerful and sought-after medicine in the world. Those who are already active, however, know they feel better after exercise. I've known for years that there was science to back this up, but even I was astonished when I discovered the sea of evidence supporting the health benefits of exercise and running. I had to come up for breath before I was swept away.

What does it mean to be fit? Physical fitness refers to the interplay between the power, endurance, and strength of skeletal muscles, the endurance of the cardiorespiratory system, flexibility, agility, reaction time, balance, and body composition.[4] All of the body's many components must come together for a body to be physically fit. You can be strong, or you can have endurance, or you can be fast. To be a long-distance runner, you need cardiorespiratory endurance, which is the ability of the circulatory and respiratory systems to supply oxygen during sustained physical exertion.[5]

There is a strong correlation between low cardiorespiratory fitness and the danger of suffering illness and premature death. Epidemiological evidence shows that low fitness increases the risk of heart disease, hypertension, stroke, metabolic syndrome, type 2 diabetes, breast and colon cancer, depression, and a person's overall risk of death.[6]

Consider the effects of exercise on the body, starting at the top and moving down. First: the brain. One of the leading causes of death in the world is the *cerebrovascular accident* (CVA), which we have come to call a *stroke*. Hippocrates first recognized stroke 2,400 years ago. The term in Greek was *apoplexy*, which means "struck down by violence." In the mid-1600s, Johann Jakob Wepfer found that patients who died with apoplexy had bleeding in the brain as well as blockages in the blood vessels of the brain. Today we recognize that strokes can involve hemorrhage, or *ischemia*. Ischemic strokes are caused by blocked or damaged vessels; these vessels can also give way, which results in catastrophic hemorrhagic strokes, in which blood pours untrammelled into the brain.

Running significantly reduces the risk of stroke. In an assessment of almost thirty thousand male runners and twelve thousand female runners followed for nearly eight years, running reduced the risk of stroke by 12 percent in men and 11 percent in women *for every kilometre run per day*. Thus, the effects kept getting bigger the farther the study subjects ran. For example, those who ran more than eight kilometres per day on average had a 60 percent lower risk of stroke than those who ran less than two kilometres per day. This study controlled for age, smoking, diabetes, high cholesterol, high blood pressure, and body mass index (BMI).[7]

The muscle impacted by all forms of exercise is the heart. If we think of the body as a beautiful machine, like a vintage convertible, it seems to follow that it would age most gracefully resting in a garage. But unlike a vintage car, the body responds to stress by getting stronger, which is why exercise has also been shown time and again to be good for cardiovascular health. The question is how much is enough. And is there such as thing as too much?

One day during lecture, a friend of mine named Adam asked our cardiology instructor, "Why does the stress of exercise make the heart stronger, while the stress of high blood pressure or myocardial infarction leads to worsening and disastrous cardiac function?" This is the miracle and mystery of exercise. We apply regular and intense stresses to our body and, for the most part, end up with a better-adapted and stronger body at the macro, organ, and cellular levels.

The benefits to the heart and the goal of preventing heart attacks led to the modern phenomenon of jogging. It began in New Zealand with a group of men in the 1960s who came to call themselves the Auckland Joggers Club.[8] It's hard to imagine what a departure this was from normal behaviour at the time. The sight of a solitary runner out, particularly at night, was treated with considerable suspicion at first. Running historian Thor Gotaas explains the prevailing wisdom of the 1950s and early 1960s: "Why would mentally healthy and law-abiding citizens bother to go running along the streets, and in the dark?"[9] In fact, one runner was arrested while out at night even after explaining that he was running for the good of his health.

Things are dramatically different today, particularly in countries that celebrate running. The author and runner Malcolm Gladwell told an interviewer for *Runner's World* of going for a run in Jamaica, on his own and just for the fun of it. To his surprise, he found himself being cheered on by people on the sidewalks, in their cars — everyone. He realized that this was a country that loved running, that smiled on its runners. When I started running and would go to a new city or country to run, I was sometimes self-conscious. I would wonder if these people had ever seen a runner before, wonder how would they react? My experiences have echoed those of Gladwell; I have been greeted by smiles and the occasional thumbs-up or high-five from a fellow runner.

But in the 1960s, the concept spread slowly through New Zealand before being exported to North America by Bill Bowerman, a coach at the University of Oregon who became fascinated by the experience after a run with the Auckland Club. In 1966 Bowerman and a cardiologist named Waldo Harris wrote the first prominent treatise on the new sport. They called it *Jogging: A Physical Fitness Program for All Ages*, and it sold millions of copies. Kenneth Cooper took the phenomenon even further. Cooper worked as a military physician and became interested in measuring and improving fitness. He developed a test for endurance using a twelve-minute run and went on to direct NASA's program for the physical conditioning of astronauts. Cooper wrote *Aerobics* in 1968, a publishing phenomenon that further galvanized public interest in running for health. The number of joggers in the United States shot up from one hundred thousand in the year *Aerobics* was published to twenty-seven million by 1977 to over forty million today.

Many factors have driven this running epidemic. It's likely, though, that knowledge of the health benefits of the sport was not one of the key ones — it's hard to get forty million people to do something hard just by telling them it's healthy. The fact that running is fun, easy to do, and feels good was probably much more important. But as the number of regular runners has grown, so has our understanding of the health benefits of running and exercise.

A decade before *Aerobics* was published, a 1953 study discovered that drivers of public trolleys in London had twice as many heart attacks as did conductors of those same trolleys. The essential difference between the two groups was that conductors walked as they collected tickets, while drivers sat for most of their workday.[10] This germinal research gave rise to the link in many scientists' minds between physical activity and the prevention of disease.[11]

More recent evidence confirms that running, in particular, reduces the risk of dying from heart disease. A study of fifty-five thousand people found that when compared to non-runners, runners were 45 percent less likely to die from cardiovascular causes. Runners had an overall *30 percent lower risk of dying* from any cause compared to non-runners, leading to an average *of three years longer lifespan.* Keep in mind that this is an average that lumps together people who run once a week with people who train for ultramarathons. Nonetheless, the results study seem to suggest that not running was, for study participants, nearly as big a risk factor for cardiovascular death as high blood pressure — it accounted for one in four cardiovascular deaths.

Another study, looking at 250,000 men and women between the ages of fifty and seventy-one, found a *50 percent reduction* in death rates in those who did vigorous exercise for sixty minutes a week and moderate exercise for another two hours per week.

I frequently discuss the subject of heart health with patients in my clinic. I enter my patient's blood pressure and cholesterol levels into a computerized tool called a Framingham Calculator, then check off if they are smokers, have diabetes, or are on blood pressure medication. Right away the patient is given a risk score. This can be a frightening experience for people, as it tells them their ten-year risk of having a heart attack. When a patient's risk is high — over 20 percent — they are usually shocked, upset. The calculator is, in a sense, a digital crystal ball, an algorithm that spells out their destiny.

It's similar to sequencing your genome to assess your risk for rare and serious conditions. This is a step that most people, including myself, hesitate to undertake. If you had your genome checked and were told you had a significant chance of developing a serious disease in the next ten years, it would be a hard fact to swallow.

Those who are high risk on the Framingham Calculator can do a few simple things to bring that risk down. The quickest way for a smoker to get the risk down is to quit smoking. Taking cholesterol or blood pressure medications can help. And then there is exercise.

The Framingham Calculator was developed using the results of the Framingham Heart Study, a massive undertaking that looked at the health of people in Framingham, Massachusetts. The study teased out what factors lead to cardiac events and death. This study has shown that an active fifty-year-old man will gain *3.7 years of life* if he is in the high exercise group and 1.3 years of life if he is in the moderate exercise group as compared to sedentary men of the same age. That is a lot of extra life.[12]

There are some facts we cannot change. A vital component of Framingham risk is family history. In fact, if your parents or siblings have significant heart disease before age fifty-five, your Framingham score is doubled.

Every time I used to go to the indoor track or to a spinning class at my local gym, I would see Andrew, a fellow physician whom I have worked with over the years. I was shocked when he told me he was seventy, as his perfect skin and muscular physique led me to believe he was at least twenty years younger. I thought that, like many doctors, he exercised because he understood the underlying benefits. Recently though, he told me he needed to go back to his cardiologist for more stenting procedures. "It's my family history," he told me. All three of his brothers had died of heart attacks in their early forties. "The only reason I've made it this long is because I've controlled my risk factors, because I'm here working out." My image of him changed instantly. For the first time, I could see the secret war he had been waging against fate.

The National Runners' Health Study has followed 120,000 runners since 1991. This study has provided a lot of the evidence that more and faster running is better. For example, speeding up your 10K time from fifty-three minutes to forty minutes could lower your risk of heart attack by about 50 percent.[13] Speed really does matter. Another study showed the speed at which a man or woman in their forties or fifties can run a mile very closely predicts their risk of heart disease in their seventies and eighties.

Cardiologists have compared a potential *polypill* with the real benefits of exercise. A polypill is a theoretical pill that could include a blood pressure medication, a medicine that protects the kidney, a cholesterol-lowering medication, and aspirin — all in one pill. Could every human benefit from such a formulation? In 2001 a group of experts concluded that such a pill could potentially improve population health.[14] But when cardiology researchers compared the polypill to exercise, they found that exercise would lead to similar reductions in blood pressure and to better improvements in healthy body weight, cardiorespiratory fitness, and superior overall health effects. Exercise is not just better than a pill; it's better than four pills.

But if exercise is a medicine, what is the right dose? Nearly all studies show that when you go from a completely sedentary life to some exercise, you get a lot of health benefits. But there may be diminishing returns. The more you do, the more benefits you receive — but only up to a point. In fact, there may come a point where a very active person may have little to no reduction in the risk of death over a sedentary person. That's not to say they don't feel better or age more gracefully; it just means they don't necessarily live much longer than less active people.

The Harvard Alumni Health Study reported a slightly higher death rate in individuals who participated in vigorous sports for more than three hours per week compared with less than three hours per week. Another study showed that patients with heart disease who did high doses of physical activity (defined as more than thirty miles per week of running and more than forty-six miles per week of walking) ended up with no benefit in terms of reduced rate of death from heart attacks, compared to people who did not exercise.[15] Another large study found no additional mortality benefits for people who engaged in more than fifty minutes per day of vigorous intensity activities.[16]

This should make us stop and think. Can too much exercise cause harm? Can exercise kill? The evidence is clear: When a healthy person follows a scientifically based training plan and listens to their body, they can put in a whole lot of training and still live to tell the tale. The life expectancy of people who exercise for up to five hours per day, every day, is no shorter than that of sedentary people.[17] Running a marathon or ultramarathon or completing an extra-long triathlon such as an Ironman is not dangerous for most people. While that may be the truth, stories of people collapsing and dying while running a race receive a great deal of media attention. These stories can inspire a fear of endurance sports. This fear can also arise if we know someone who has experienced a medical emergency while running. During the 2008 Berlin Marathon, the twenty-five-year-old Congolese Canadian marathoner Danny Kassap collapsed; he survived only because a spectator immediately performed CPR. He was placed in a medically induced coma and found to have a cardiac dysrhythmia resulting from some sort of cardiac inflammation. He was able to return to running, but he ended up dying three years later in Toronto the day after withdrawing from another race.

The number of marathon finishers in the United States has risen from twenty-five thousand in 1976 to over half a million in recent years, while nearly two million people complete a half-marathon each year. Among all these runners, about one in one hundred thousand runners die of sudden cardiac death during a marathon, and one in four hundred thousand runners die in a half-marathon.[18] While the overall rate is very low, people do die. That risk of death of one in one hundred thousand compares to a 1.5 in one hundred thousand risk of dying while participating in a triathlon and one in one million risk of dying during a year of regular swimming.

The cardiologists and exercise researchers who were concerned about the harms of exercise suggested that too much endurance activity could cause cardiac arrhythmias and damage to the precious muscle of the heart known as the myocardium.[19] When someone has a heart attack, the level of a chemical called cardiac troponin in their blood shoots up. Up to one third of runners tested after marathons have elevated levels of cardiac troponin. Also, imaging studies show increases in the size of the atria — the upper chambers of the heart through which blood enters before being pumped out — and worse cardiac function in the hearts of runners immediately after a marathon. But all the cardiac abnormalities resolve after one to three days and no obvious long-term damage is seen in the hearts of most marathoners.[20] People also walk funny and hurt all over after a marathon, but no one is worried they will walk funny and hurt forever.

Many deaths during marathons and other extreme events are in individuals with the rare condition known as idiopathic *hypertrophic cardiomyopathy*. This is a condition wherein the left ventricle of the heart is excessively large, usually due to a mutation in the genes coding for part of the pumping region of the heart. The condition is found in one in two hundred adults and usually causes few or no symptoms, but the abnormality can be picked up on electrocardiogram (ECG) or by an ultrasound of the heart, known as an echocardiogram. On average, individuals with this condition have a normal life expectancy. A few, however, are predisposed to develop cardiac arrhythmias during stressful exertion, which accounts for about one third of the cases of sudden deaths during marathons.

But while the evidence is clear that there is no such thing as too much exercise, we still seem to face the Goldilocks problem — finding just the right dose of exercise. The studies of the "extreme" exercisers, men and women who go for five hours a day, don't seem to show them having any mortality benefits over people who are just meeting the minimum dose of thirty minutes per day. The perfect dose would help a person feel great, look great, and live as long as possible. The perfect dose would also be the one with the fewest side effects, such as overuse injuries, which can completely sideline your ability to exercise for a time.

One way of looking at the optimal dosage of exercise needed was provided in 2016 by the Global Burden of Disease Study.[21] To understand this study, you need to understand the concept of the MET, or metabolic equivalent of task. The MET is a measure that expresses the energy cost of a physical activity. One MET is the energy you might expend while seated at rest. More intense forms of exercise are worth more METs. Intensive aerobic activity might be equivalent of six or more METs, meaning that six times more energy is expended than would normally be expended sitting doing nothing.

The World Health Organization and many other governments and agencies want us to aim for 150 minutes of moderate-intensity activity per week. This amount of activity is calculated to be an average of six hundred MET minutes of total activity per week. For the Global Burden of Disease Study, the authors looked at the link between the total number of MET minutes people logged per week and five outcomes: breast cancer, colon cancer, diabetes, ischemic heart disease, and ischemic stroke.

What was different about this study is that it did not just include scheduled exercise like running; it included all activity expended throughout the day, including walking up and down stairs, cleaning, putting away the laundry, cooking — everything. And what they found was that more activity per week is better — a lot more. Some activity was better than none, and the gains kept on growing as people were more and more active. Most of the gains occurred at a total activity level of three thousand to four thousand MET minutes per week. This is five to seven times more than the currently recommended six hundred MET minutes per week. This translates into 750 to 1,050 minutes per week of moderate-intensity exercise, which could mean as much as 2.5 hours per day of moderate-intensity exercise every day of the year.

The authors give an example of how you could achieve three thousand MET minutes per week, it would involve "climbing the stairs for ten minutes, vacuuming for fifteen minutes, gardening for twenty minutes, running for twenty minutes, then walking or cycling for transportation for twenty-five minutes."[22] With this example, in ninety minutes a day, you could get the minimum three thousand MET minutes per week. Achieving four thousand would take even more work.

I think this is an important study in this field because it is so comprehensive, looking at all types of activity. It may be correct that you only need to run twenty minutes a day to achieve optimal health benefits — but that's true only if you incorporate another seventy minutes of activity into your day.

In the summer of 2019 a group of Scandinavian exercise researchers provided another answer to the question of the right dose.[23] The researchers took forty-eight studies, which together included over eight hundred thousand participants, and looked for the association between weekly duration of exercise and the risk of death. The results were impressive. The risk of death dropped quickly as people went from no activity to low levels, then reached the lowest point at about two thousand MET minutes per week, or about four hours of moderate-intensity exercise a week. The overall risk then slowly climbed afterward, but it never went up to the same level as for inactive people. And it wasn't heart disease that was causing problems for people at higher levels of activity. In fact, the risk of any kind of heart disease kept going down as activity levels went up.

To try to make sense of the swirl of confusing ideas around the ideal dose of exercise, I went to Toronto to meet with Alex Hutchinson. I had been following Hutchinson's writing on exercise science for almost as long as I'd been a runner. He had made a name for himself as a translator of exercise science, and everyone in the running community waited with great anticipation for his 2018 book *Endure: Mind, Body, and the Curiously Elastic Limits of Human Performance* to come out. When it did arrive, it was a sensation and his standing as a guru of running science rose even higher.

I flew to Toronto early in the morning in mid-January and watched as the snow-covered landscape of Ontario passed below me. I was wearing my trail running shoes and my running outfit was stuffed into my backpack along with my sunglasses and a couple bananas. It had been extremely cold for the past week, but things had warmed up to around zero on this day.

When Hutchinson arrived at our meeting point, he was dressed for winter running with a black tuque and running gloves. We chatted for a moment and then Hutchinson and I were off, running the trails of High Park. I immediately noticed Hutchinson's controlled running technique. He seemed to be taking perfectly efficient steps as he began to lead me on one of his regular training routes. He told me he does most of his running along the Humber River, but High Park was a good place to come in winter and was close to his home.

He knew I had come to talk about mortality and exercise dose, and he didn't waste any time. He told me he didn't have much faith in the big cohort studies because there were just too many variables that couldn't all be controlled for. He told me about a paper by Daniel Lieberman, which argues that there is no perfect evolutionary dose of exercise. I had read the paper years ago but forgotten that was one of the central messages. Alex made a lot of other good points, but as I was breathing heavily and couldn't stop to take notes, some of the details were lost. This was my first attempt at doing journalism while running, and I realized I still had a few kinks to work out.

We ran through the bright winter morning alongside the frozen expanse of Grenadier Pond, occasionally pausing on an icy patch. Then we took a long path uphill and I felt my breathing coming faster. I paced myself as I tried to make intelligent responses to Hutchinson's exposition. Finally, mercifully, he turned around and we stopped running.

Hutchinson and I walked back to the restaurant where we had met and ordered lunch. I felt flushed by the run through the cold morning and happy to be talking to someone who was so knowledgeable about running and so willing to share his knowledge. We talked about the running books we liked, about human exploration, about the idea of nature, and about our kids. Soon it was time for me to go to another meeting and for Hutchinson to get back to his life. We said our goodbyes, and I went and changed out of my running clothes back into my civilian outfit.

Later that afternoon I flew back to Ottawa, knowing that I had added another thread to my running history, without necessarily having cracked the secret of the perfect dose of exercise. But I had been reassured that it's hard — if not impossible — to get too much of this particular good thing. And we don't just do things because they make us live longer; we are motivated by many factors.

Beyond changes to the heart and life expectancy, there is the effect of exercise on body weight, another topic that Hutchinson and I touched upon. Early humans were faced with the constant struggle to stay on the positive side of energy balance; today, 70 percent (more than two out of every three) of Americans are overweight or obese compared to 63 percent of Canadians. More than 50 percent of Europeans are overweight or obese. Rates of obesity and its concomitant diseases are also increasing in India, China, and virtually every other country on the planet.

It is very hard to lose weight. I once trained with an endocrinologist in a women's health clinic. We met a patient trying to lose weight. She listed all the changes she had made in her diet and all the physical activity she had added to her life. Through tears, she told us how little she had to show in terms of weight loss for all the efforts she had made. The endocrinologist sympathized with her: "The brain is a very sophisticated computer, and if it doesn't want you to lose weight, it's very hard to do so."

That notion stuck with me, and when I saw a recent study that followed participants in the reality TV show *The Biggest Loser*, her words came back to me. The study tracked the participants after the show to see whether they were able to maintain their weight loss. The brutal reality is that they didn't. Most gained back at least 50 percent of what they had lost, and some even ended up heavier than before. Was this because they lacked the willpower to maintain the healthy changes they had made under the bright lights of reality TV? No. As was the case with our patient in the women's health clinic, their brains had changed the rules of the game to try to get them back to their original weight. Most participants had metabolic rates far slower than they should have, given their weight, age, and sex. Somewhere in the hormonal control centre, a warning light was flashing, alerting the body of weight loss and doing everything to regain that weight.

A follow-up study from 2017 looked in more detail at those who were able to maintain considerable weight loss — eighty-one pounds on average — after six years.[24] As the original study had found, the participants' metabolisms slowed dramatically, resulting in their bodies burning five hundred fewer calories per day than would be expected. The few who did maintain their weight loss massively increased their moderate physical activity to eighty minutes per day in order to counter this slowed metabolism. Importantly, these eighty minutes weren't dedicated to exercise alone; the time included all activities such as walking briskly and housecleaning.

The questions persist: Why does the brain want to get the body back to its *highest* weight? Why not the ideal weight? We don't have that answer yet. What we do know is that while our brains are supercomputers in some ways, they can also be dumb computers, reacting to hormones and stimuli in ways that are actually harmful to our bodies. Again, this goes back to the caveman hypothesis. As Daniel Lieberman argues, there would have been no situation in prehistory when too many calories would have been a problem. Similarly, there would have been no time when too little physical activity would have been a problem either. Like climate change, these problems are products of human invention, and we must now invent our way out of them. Medical solutions will likely be developed that allow us to block or manipulate the brain's resistance to weight loss. This will be a boon to those currently suffering from obesity. For everyone else, the focus should remain on prevention.

Runners weigh less than non-runners. Multiple large studies have shown runners' BMI is one to two points less than non-runners'. An increase in the intensity of exercise leads to more benefit. A very large study found a BMI of 25.2 in those who run the least per week and 23.9 in those who run the most, compared to 26.3 in non-runners. In those trying to lose weight, people who improve their diet and exercise have more reduction in body fat compared to people who change only their diet.[25]

More exercise also reduces the risk of high blood pressure, high cholesterol, and type 2 diabetes. A study of over thirty thousand runners and over fifteen thousand walkers found that both running and walking were associated with a reduced risk for high blood pressure, high cholesterol, and type 2 diabetes. The fittest men in the study had a reduction of 62 percent in high blood pressure, 67 percent in high cholesterol, and 86 percent less type 2 diabetes compared to the least fit group of men. Running more marathons per year has also been shown to reduce the prevalence of all three conditions.

The first time I was asked to read an X-ray in front of my classmates, I saw the white grooves of the femoral condyle reaching down to meet the tibial plateau — it was a knee. "What features of osteoarthritis does this image demonstrate?" the radiology resident asked in a distant voice. This was too routine to be interesting to him, but my hands were sweating. The knee did not look healthy. I mumbled something about the joint space looking narrow; the normally well-formed lines of the joint space had been replaced by a jagged sclerotic mess where bone met bone. Then

I saw the small white dots — osteophytes — the bony spurs that form in arthritic bone. I can still see that X-ray now when I feel the grinding crepitus of an elderly patient's sore knee.

A common concern raised about running is its impact on the knee and on a runner's overall risk of osteoarthritis. In fact, the evidence shows that running is protective against arthritis. A 2013 study of seventy-five thousand runners showed that there is no evidence linking any type of running to knee osteoarthritis, not even marathon running. Runners were actually less likely to develop arthritis than non-runners. Other studies have shown that running and walking, but not other types of exercise, provide an equal reduction in osteoarthritis and in the risk of needing a hip replaced at some point in your life.[26]

This finding goes against the common-sense notion that more use leads to more wear and tear. How could the opposite be true? For one thing, running leads to lower a BMI, and higher BMI is a risk factor for osteoarthritis. Another study compared running with walking and found that while runners hit the ground with eight times their body weight, they took fewer strides and had shorter impact times compared to walkers. In the end, this led to an equal stress on the knees for walkers and runners.

Osteoarthritis is getting much more common. In 2017 Daniel Lieberman's group looked at the knees of prehistoric skeletons and knees from the 1800s and compared them to modern knees. They found that only 8 percent of prehistoric skeletons had knee osteoarthritis compared to 6 percent of knees from the 1800s, whereas 16 percent of more recent knees had the disease, even after controlling for age, body mass index, and other factors.

Lieberman's group uses this finding to argue that aging and rising BMI — the usual culprits — are not enough to explain this rising prevalence. Instead, they point the finger at physical inactivity. Weaker joints are more susceptible to damage. If you use your joints less as children, you develop thinner cartilage. Less musculature around the joint provides less stabilization and increases the force experienced in the joint. Finally, inflammation, which can be worsened by a diet replete with highly refined carbohydrates, may be making things even worse. They conclude with a call to arms: "It is likely that any effective prevention strategy will involve adjusting physical activity patterns and diets to approximate more closely the lifestyle conditions under which our species evolved."[27]

More exercise protects the joints and leads to stronger bones. Weight-bearing exercise promotes the growth of new bone, leading to an increase in bone mineral density in both men and women. Even patients who already have osteoporosis are at decreased risk of hip fracture if they exercise regularly.[28]

As I mentioned earlier, exercise also reduces your risk of colon and breast cancer. In fact, physical activity may provide protection against breast, kidney, intestinal, prostate, endometrial, brain, and pancreatic cancer. In a meta-analysis that looked at twenty-one studies, the most active people had 27 percent less colon cancer compared to those who were least active.[29]

The biggest risk factor for cancer is aging, and people tend to exercise less as they get older. During my own fellowship training, I took a special interest in HIV and aging, for the simple fact that the global population is aging, and the face of the HIV epidemic is becoming older every year. More than 50 percent of HIV positive individuals in North America are now over fifty years of age. Through studying this connection, I came to discover the scientific study of aging. I became fascinated by the question of why we age. One night, after a long run, I went to a talk where the speaker showed a *Time* magazine cover with a picture of a baby and the headline, "This Baby Could Live to be 142 Years Old." For decades, life expectancy increased year after year, until in recent years things have slowed down and even reversed in North America while continuing to climb to ever-higher levels in Japan.

Humanity is aging. The median age will increase from twenty-seven in 2000 to forty-six by the year 2100. Over this century, the proportion of the global population over sixty will grow from one in ten to one in three. The population over eighty-five years old has been the fastest growing segment of the population in industrialized countries.[30] Humans are living longer. Are they also living better?

Aging is the progressive deterioration in the body's function resulting from a lifetime of molecular, cellular, and organ damage.[31] Aging occurs in part because of the cumulative damage to your DNA but also from a progressive decline in cellular function. Free radicals fly off like sparks during the operation of our molecular machinery, and these sparks damage our DNA. Failing cells start to build up in our organs. Errors creep into our software.

Aging also results in more exercise-related injuries. The injury rate climbs steeply in competitive runners over the age of fifty. One reason is thought to be the degradation of collagen in connective tissues. Patients are always incredulous when they come to me, usually in their fifties, and say, "But doctor I've never been sick/injured/tired like this before." After looking into possible causes, I usually need to gently remind them that their age, while out of their control, is part of the problem.

A key aspect of aging is that it results in the extra length at the end of our DNA, called telomeres, becoming shorter with each cell replication until there's nothing left. Telomeres keep chromosomes stable.[32] They are the extra buttons that come with your new trousers, and once you use them up, you don't have any more buttons. Shortening telomeres are associated with numerous chronic diseases across a spectrum of ages.[33]

There are only a few ways to live longer. Calorie restriction seems to be one of them. Reducing caloric intake by 30 percent seems to lead to about 40 percent extension of lifespan in animal models. This may be due to less metabolism leading to less oxidative damage to cells. And then of course there is exercise. I tell those patients of mine who are incredulous about getting injured as they age about the importance of exercise to mitigate these effects. Aerobic fitness has been shown to be a better predictor of longevity than any other health measurement.[34]

We have already seen that exercise reduces a host of diseases and can add extra years of life. Regular physical activity can actually *lengthen* telomeres, which explains one mechanism by which exercise leads to a longer life. A 2010 study looked at telomere length in young and old active and sedentary subjects. Both the active and inactive young groups had similar telomere lengths, but the older inactive group had much shorter telomeres compared to their contemporaries who had put in at least forty-five minutes of vigorous exercise five times a week.[35] Another study comparing pairs of identical twins found longer telomeres in the more active of the twins.[36]

A fascinating study by Paul D. Loprinzi and Eveleen Sng looked at this finding in more detail and made a surprising discovery. The investigators created a model incorporating age, sex, ethnicity, weight, total cholesterol, a marker of inflammation, monthly amounts of physical activity, and whether individuals met nine different physical activity guidelines.[37] The model showed that the only type of physical activity that was significantly associated with the lengthening of telomeres was, you guessed it, running.

Loprinzi and Sng were as surprised by this finding as I was when I read the paper while sitting at my kitchen counter one sunny morning. The authors point out these findings match other studies that have shown, for example, that ultramarathon runners have longer telomeres than healthy individuals from the general population. What's more, longer telomere length is associated with both lower rates of cardiovascular disease and lower death rates, both of which have been found to be benefits of regular running.

Loprinzi and Sng hypothesized why this may be. Exercise leads to changes in signalling pathways that are linked to telomere biology and form. It is possible that the sustained weight bearing generated when running may be "optimal in activating these signalling pathways."[38] We don't yet know why telomeres lengthen in runners, but we have good evidence that it is happening. Murakami observes in his running memoir, "I'll be happy if running and I can grow old together." It certainly appears that the two can go nicely together. In fact, many of the changes thought to be associated with aging are actually consequences of physical inactivity.[39]

Exercise even has an anti-aging effect at the molecular level. Another fascinating study looked at what happens to stem cells, the basic type of cell that can grow into a variety of different types of cells, when submitted to exercise-like stresses. Whereas most stem cells will turn into fat cells, cells that are stimulated with forces equivalent to jogging can be coaxed to transform into bone cells. The scientist who conducted this study said, "This is the first time in my career that something I've done in the lab has changed how I work out."[40]

You live longer and better if you are more active. The loss of muscle mass as we age — *sarcopenia* — can be substantially slowed by regular exercise. For millennia, humans have aspired to be "super-agers," to remain young in mind and body long after other people start to show signs of deterioration and decay.[41] In legend and myth, this is achieved through potions and dark magic. Herculean exercise is more likely to work. One of the keys to becoming a "super-ager" is to push your body and mind to the point of pain. You can't do something easy like running the same thirty-minute loop every day; you need to push the pace or push the distance or try a new sport or learn a new language and struggle to achieve your goal. The super-ager concept reflects the United States Marine Corps mantra: "Pain is weakness leaving your body."

A key feature of aging is declining cognitive function. One day in clinic I was reading the news in between patients, and I came across a study linking leg strength to cognitive function. What made the study particularly powerful was the fact that it compared twins, reviewed their leg strength over time, and connected this to their performance on cognitive tests. The leg muscles are the largest muscles in the body, and muscular power is seen as a marker of healthy aging. The study found that twins who had more muscular power, over time, performed significantly better on memory and cognitive tests and had less brain atrophy than their weaker siblings. The study concluded by positing that interventions that allow people to improve leg power may help society reach a goal of "healthy cognitive aging."[42]

Exercise has been shown to particularly benefit brain activities involving executive control, such as planning, monitoring, and task coordination.[43] And it's never too late to start exercising. A small mountain of evidence shows that the benefits to muscle, the cardiovascular system, and the brain can be experienced by people even if they start exercising in old age after a relatively sedentary life.[44]

But how can health care providers help patients exercise more? One morning in my clinic I counselled Chris, a patient who had previously been a very successful cyclist. In his early sixties at the time, he was overweight, pre-diabetic, and suffering from high cholesterol. He had knee and back pain. I knew that exercise would help with all of these problems. I asked him why he wasn't active, and he told me he had given up cycling and other exercise years ago as the demands of his desk job took over his time. I talked to him about why he should change — cited statistics about the reduction in his risk of diabetes, heart disease, stroke, cancer, dementia, and more. He listened quietly, looking guilty. He told me he knew he needed to change, he wanted to change, but he couldn't find the motivation.

As I was running by the river later at lunchtime, I thought about Chris and a theme that runs through all my medical practice: What's the best way to make patients change their behaviours? One patient continued to drink too much, despite all the standard treatments we tried. Another patient refused to take his blood thinners, despite having a clot lodged in his heart. And so many others could not be motivated to exercise.

The first step is to ask about the behaviours. Studies have shown that less than one third of patients in primary care clinics report getting advice from their physicians about physical activity. Physicians can assess the amount of physical activity as a *vital sign* and provide an exercise prescription based on that vital sign. In recognition of this approach, a large international movement called *Exercise Is Medicine* began in 2007. It works with physicians, exercise professionals, university campuses, and the public to promote evidence-based knowledge about physical activity.

My clinic took up the baton a few years ago and added the physical activity vital sign (PAVS) to our triage procedure for every patient. It's quite simple: each time a patient comes to the clinic, they are given a tablet to check their contact information and health card. We added a routine question about smoking. If they are smokers, the tablet asks them how much they are smoking and whether they would be ready to engage in a cessation program at that clinic visit. These questions need to be answered before each visit, ensuring that smoking status never drops off the agenda of the patient or their doctor.

Using the same logic, we added the PAVS to each clinic visit. So now when I sit down with a patient, their electronic chart has been updated to include the number of minutes they exercise each week. The goal is at least 150, and if they typically record less than that number, they are prompted to discuss ways to improve their exercise routine with their doctor. As with noting their smoking, completing the PAVS reminds patients that exercise is a critical part of their health that should be at or near the top of the agenda at each clinic visit.

Once we know their physical activity vital sign, we try to assess their readiness to change. If, like Chris, they want to change, we can use a range of tools. Virtually every strategy has been tried. Early traditional healers would harness supernatural authorities to promote change. Then, for the longest time, physicians relied on their personal charisma to inspire others to follow their commandments, even though so much advice was useless at best and dangerous at worst. More recently, physicians have used science as the weapon with which to change behaviour. Often this works, especially if we can link risk to the patient's specific issue. To show someone a graph of their blood sugar trending up over time can be a powerful motivator for change.

But the new approach to behaviour change aims to be subtler and is premised on the idea that if you push patients and use fear tactics, they push back and use denial to quell their fears. Saying something like, "If you keep smoking, you will die of lung disease" often leads someone to retort, "I like smoking and my grandmother lived to eighty-seven and smoked every day of her life." Teachers of motivational interviewing advise that it's best to begin a discussion by eliciting information from the person being interviewed. For example, when discussing their smoking habit with a patient, I will start by getting them to tell me their thoughts about smoking: "Tell me what you like and what you don't like about smoking." Patients are usually so shocked that you want to hear a list of the good things about smoking that they let their guard down. You help them explore their motivations for change and build on that. You don't push; you nudge and let them take the initiative.

Some days I am a 1950s doctor, wielding facts and knowledge from on high, educating patients about the mental and physical effects of alcohol abuse or listing the effects of marijuana on a fetus. Other days I sit quietly in my swivel chair and let my patients open up to me about the feelings they have when they use cocaine, how angry they are with themselves, and how much they hate to use cocaine, and with only a few words from me, they have themselves decided on the new steps they will take to stop using drugs.

Studies have explored whether health care providers can actually make a difference to their patients' exercise levels. Large reviews show that exercise counselling does make a difference to patients' level of activity but may make less difference to objective outcomes like physical fitness. Counselling alone isn't usually enough. We need to be creative with our patients. Workplace strategies like standing desks and walking desks can reduce sitting time, although standing has its own issues. Encouraging people to get up and out of their chair every thirty to sixty minutes and walk for up to five minutes helps people stay awake and gives much needed activity.

When I was a medical student at SickKids Hospital in Toronto, there were signs encouraging employees to take the stairs or, as they had been renamed, the "Stairway to Health." I loved this idea. I was further convinced of the wisdom of such marketing when I saw a study about a program that encouraged hospital volunteers to take the stairs instead of the elevator for six weeks. In that short time, they found the volunteers had lower blood pressure, lower weight, and improved cholesterol.

Using pedometers, activity monitors such as Fitbits, and smart watches can also help. A systematic review of traditional pedometers found that people walk more if they wear one. If wearers were given a goal of a certain numbers of steps per day — usually set at ten thousand steps — the pedometers led to 27 percent more activity, and also resulted in lower BMI and lower blood pressure. More people, including many friends of mine, are becoming voluntarily enslaved to their smart watches. Some devices periodically remind their wearers to get up and move and chastise them at the end of each day if they have not met their physical activity goals. This is powerful technology and is rapidly advancing.

One day a young man who had been suffering from chronic neck and lower back pain came to my office smiling and told me he felt better. "What's changed?" I asked him. He had started the "7-minute workout" using an app on his phone. He told me how the app motivated him to do intense, thirty-second bursts of eleven different exercises with ten-second breaks between. "I can barely move by the end of it, but since I've started doing it, I've been feeling better." I had read about the workout and had been meaning to try it, so his story motivated me to buy the three-dollar app and give it a try.

The next day I set up my workout mat in my office and turned on the app, and I was immediately hooked. The intensity of the exercise and the blending of upper and lower body exercises offered a refreshing contrast to running. I did three cycles the first day and kept doing it every day for the next week. I developed a routine involving a run to a nearby pedestrian bridge, doing my seven minutes out in the open, then running back to my office. Within days, I felt stronger, and I was grateful to the young patient who had motivated me to begin the new routine.

The higher-intensity training studies and regimes keep coming. The Tabata method involves alternating twenty-second periods of activity with ten seconds of rest for four minutes. Another, the "1-minute workout," involves sixty seconds of intense cycling with nine minutes of slow cycling. Incredibly, studies show that these workouts produce impressive and often superior results compared to longer periods of exercise, and it's easier to get someone to commit to seven minutes of exercise than it is to persuade them to train for an ultramarathon.

I remember when my younger brother told me about the running app that had got him running. I used that same app the next day, and it rekindled my passion for running. More and more, we are seeing the potential of the apps that we can download onto the smartphones we all carry to change our behaviour.

Technology has a role, as does social pressure. Running or training with a group leads to more consistency and higher intensity, and also provides immense social benefits. I have been following with interest the science of happiness and well-being. Some long-term studies, such as the Harvard Study of Adult Development, have shown that strong relationships and feelings of social connection are critical for maintaining health. Socializing while exercising provides a happy synergy. Personal trainers have also been shown to improve motivation, and a trainer can make a huge difference to people who do not know how to exercise safely.

But many of the strategies to increase physical activity need planning and investment from government and businesses. Having showers and bike parking at an office encourages active commuting. Having safe paths for runners and bikers is also vital. Reducing suburban sprawl and building walkable neighbourhoods centred around public transport also helps. Taking the bus has been shown to provide more exercise than commuting by car. Such changes pay for themselves: improving the health of people reduces the number of sick days taken by employees and, more importantly, reduces the burden placed on the medical system.

A huge number of studies have examined the benefits and potential risks of exercise. One day, thinking about these hundreds of studies, I stopped for a moment and asked myself, *Do I feel healthier since I started running?* I have felt different: I've felt more stable and stronger, in every sense of the word. I am a runner, and that gives me a sense of belonging.

In the next chapter, we will explore the mental aspect of running, how it calms, helps people sleep, and brings some of them, some of the time, to new heights of experience.

IV RUNNING AND MENTAL HEALTH

One day in early April I went for a long run around Hog's Back Falls and the Rideau River. A few weeks before, the paths had been impassable from snow and ice. Then the snow melted. Then it flooded. Crews were out removing the debris and large branches that had been strewn about by the flooding. Parts of my neighbourhood were under water, and on the other side of the Ottawa River, dozens of homes were evacuated despite the city deploying sixty-five thousand sandbags. At long last the water receded. Suddenly, hundreds of kilometres of running trails were released from the grip of winter, and I found myself yearning to start those long runs along the dirt trails. It is on the very longest runs that the mind and body ascend to the highest, the most transcendent states.

* * *

To my mind, running involves, in large part, being in and mindful of nature. The Swiss writer Jack Schumacher travelled to Finland in the 1930s to meet the greatest runner of the day, a Finn named Paavo Nurmi. Schumacher wrote:

> Running is in the blood of every Finn. When you see these pure, deep forests, these fertile wide-open fields with typical, red-painted workers' houses, these ridges with their clusters of trees, the endless blue horizon that shades over into lakes, then you are overwhelmed by excitement and you feel the urge to run — because we have no wings to fly. Just to run on light feet through this Nordic landscape for mile after mile and hour after hour. Nurmi and those like him are animals in the forest. They began to run because of a profound compulsion, because a strange dream-like landscape called them with its enchanting mysteries.[1]

Schumacher's mixed metaphors and purple prose captures the joys of running in nature. I remember reading E.O. Wilson's descriptions of the key features of ideal habitats across all human cultures. The three features that we tend to seek are an elevated position, a view of parkland, and, ideally, a view of water. Any of my favourite running trails includes two or three of those features.

The author Neal Bascomb describes a time in Roger Bannister's life when the great runner was struggling with his failure at the 1952 Helsinki Olympics and the relentless media pressure to perform:

> To escape the attention, he journeyed to Scotland to hike and sleep under the stars for two weeks. One late afternoon, after swimming in a lake, he began to jog around to ease his chill. Soon enough he found himself running for the sheer exhilaration of it, across the moor and toward the coast. The sky was filled with crimson clouds, and as he ran a light rain started to

> fall. With the sun still warming his back, a rainbow appeared in front of him, and he seemed to run toward it. Along the coast the rhythm of the water breaking around the rocks eased him, and he circled back to where he had begun. Cool, wet air filled his lungs.... He had needed to reconnect to the joy of running.[2]

Why do we run? Because it feels good to run. And the greatest sense of well-being is unlocked when we run outside in nature. Exercising outdoors and in natural surroundings, in particular, has greater mental health benefits than exercising indoors or in an urban environment. People who exercise in nature are also more likely to stick with fitness routines than those who exercise indoors.[3]

People who exercise in a natural setting are less anxious, experience more mood elevation, and have better cognitive performance than those who run on city streets.[4] Anyone who has run both through traffic and along a bucolic riverbank understands this. There is even evidence that patients who recover from surgery or heart attacks in rooms looking at natural settings have less depression and shorter recovery times compared to people without such views.

One researcher rhetorically asks us to "imagine a therapy that had no known side effects, was readily available, and could improve your cognitive functioning at zero cost." That therapy is interacting with nature.[5] Look around your home or office, and you will probably find plants, images of natural settings, or a screensaver portraying a churning ocean. Even without knowing the evidence, we gravitate toward nature.

So it is with exercise. Whenever I talk to patients about coping with stress, we look at ways to get more outdoor time, more walks or runs along the river, more time cycling through the forest, more swimming. The writer Moriel Rothman-Zecher wrote a beautiful account of his brother's recovery from a bicycle accident. Rothman-Zecher flew to California to be with his brother during his extended ICU and rehabilitation stay. Rothman-Zecher coped with the emotions he experienced by training for an ultramarathon, a sport he had shared with his brother. On his various runs, he had a series of surreal brushes with nature — two rattlesnakes mating, a coyote pack, a mountain lion. As his brother recovered, this distance running through untamed desert allowed Rothman-Zecher to be emotionally present for him.

All exercise, even when we work out inside while watching television, profoundly changes our mood, our ability to cope with stress, and our sleep. I began to dabble in running while trying to cope with the stress of being a medical resident — trying to think about what sort of career I envisioned for myself, worrying about exams, student debt, and coming to terms with the awesome responsibility of practising medicine on my own, outside of the comforting cocoon of med school and residency. This dabbling led to me to train for my first race after my reincarnation as a runner. I trained predominantly at night after my son had gone to bed. I left the house with my wife curled up reading on the couch and headed out into the quiet night.

On weekends I aimed for longer distances. One Sunday morning, I ran from my house along the canal, around Dow's Lake, and back home. It was a distance of around eight kilometres, which, at the time, felt momentous. I came back babbling with excitement, telling my family about the great distance I had travelled, the red-winged blackbirds I had seen swooping low over fellow runners, and the euphoria. The euphoria was bliss. The remainder of the day I played with my son and enjoyed feeling so alive.

On race day there was a complication. I was actually on call for the hospital all weekend, so I would need to run with my cellphone and answer any calls during the race. I informed my colleagues I would be a little late coming in that morning, and in the end they successfully deflected any calls from interrupting my race.

My race was only one of a dozen events held that morning, which included triathlons of every possible distance including an Ironman. I joined the small pack of about one hundred runners at the start line for the 10K. One woman wore a T-shirt with the phrase "You were just passed by a pregnant woman" on the back.

The horn sounded and I was off, racing for the first time since cross-country fifteen years earlier. Like many first-time racers, I let the competition take control and push me too fast. I more or less sprinted through the first four kilometres, staying with the leaders before realizing that I had spent nearly all my reserves. As I approached the halfway point, I began wishing I had only committed to the 5K race. I slowed to a jogging pace and prepared for the next five kilometres. Finishing the race was painful, but I managed to keep running through the second half. I debriefed with my father and my wife that night over dinner. That hot August day I was reborn as a runner.

Following that, I ran a 10K in Oka National Park. The course in Oka was a combination of trail and road. We weaved through a forest before coming out to a large road then circling back. I paced myself as I remembered the lesson of my first race. In fact, I went too slowly, and over the last three kilometres I still had a lot of energy and I pushed myself, passing dozens of runners before finishing with a respectable time. From the finish line, I walked toward the shore of the river and yelled into the trees with triumph. I felt so alive, marvelling that this was what it was all about, this was the power of racing, this was how it felt to be fast! Hours later, I returned home, tired and feeling the inner contentment that I had come to associate with racing. That night I went to sleep early, and I woke up the next morning having experienced another of the runner's joy: the peaceful post-race sleep.

Every week I spend many hours with patients working on improving their sleep. I have done extra reading on this subject and have come to realize that an epidemic of insomnia plagues our society. Patients complain of not being able to get to sleep, of getting to sleep but then waking after only three to four hours, or of waking too early. Some nap; some do not. Some are stressed about work; some have severe anxiety disorders and their minds churn restlessly as soon as they make contact with their pillows. But many say they have no extraordinary stress and are not anxious; they just can't sleep. They want to know why. They want to fix the problem.

Insomnia is a symptom that is both common and disabling. When we can't sleep, we are frustrated, cranky, anxious, unpleasant, and unable to focus or perform to the best of our abilities. When I run early-morning races, I am also anxious and restless, worried about sleeping through the alarm, worried about getting my race bib on time. I drink my one cup of coffee and arrive bleary-eyed at the race site wishing I could enjoy the experience without the extra burden of insomnia-induced fatigue. After the race I feel good, but that night I will sleep like I have been blessed by the gods. The only comparison to that rest I can think of is the sleep I had as a child after a day of playing on the beach. I ran and swam and ate hard-boiled eggs and drank juice. On the drive home, the car radio was playing softly, and the thrill of the beach began to give way to hypnagogic bobs and flights of the imagination, the prelude to dreams. Then I was home, bundled up in my bedroom, and finally, I gave myself up to sleep.

I try to evoke similar moments in my patients with insomnia. Remember childhood? Remember how sleep crept into your bed, overcoming any resistance, closing your eyes? They often do remember the sleep of childhood, and we work on returning their sleep to that innocent state. What did they know as a child that they have forgotten as an adult? Playing, the outdoors, running themselves ragged. I remind them of our evolutionary forerunners — the destiny for thousands of generations of our ancestors: running, hunting, and then sleeping peacefully in caves beside the communal fire. Of course, running is not the answer for everyone, but when they return weeks later, having turned off the television in the bedroom, stopped emailing in bed, slowly built up time outdoors for physical activity, they are sleeping better. It takes time and diligence to undo the effects of urban life and inactivity.

A study showed that it takes about four months for regular exercise to improve sleep.[6] This time lag may explain why many people don't make the connection between increased exercise and improved sleep — it doesn't happen right away. In this study participants did only thirty minutes of aerobic exercises three times per week; more intense and frequent exercise may have led to quicker results. Yet these participants slept forty-five minutes longer, had better sleep efficiency, and described better sleep quality four months after starting this program. It takes time for our background stress and anxiety, which are reinforced by neural pathways in the brain, to be dialed down. Interestingly, the relationship between sleep and exercise was *bidirectional*: better sleep leaves us feeling refreshed and leaves us with more energy, which leads to better exercise sessions. This is something that we have all experienced.

What about exercise and mood? Remember your first exercise high? Mine was after cross-country training in Cairo during the winter of grade nine. At that time, we talked about endorphins, the body's natural opioids, causing the high. The role of endorphins was confirmed in a 2008 study, in which subjects ran for two hours then had their brains assessed for endorphin levels. This study showed endorphins were released into their brains and also found that higher levels were correlated with a more intense runner's high.[7]

The relationship between exercise and mood involves more than endorphin levels, however; it is more complex. The body's cannabis system also plays a part. We know, from studies conducted with mice, that the body's own cannabis molecule, known as *anandamide*, which is produced during exercise, helps reduce anxiety and increase pain tolerance. Blocking opioid receptors in the brains of mice does not seem to block an exercise high in the same way as blocking endocannabinoid receptors does. Exercise increases anandamide levels, but persistent psychological stress actually decreases these levels. Thus, the physical stress of exercise boosts mood, while the sedentary stress of finances, work, commuting, and worries has the opposite effect.[8] And you get the most benefit from the best form of exercise, which is moderate intensity. Moderate-intensity exercise — running while still being able to talk — is the intensity that leads to steepest rise in brain endocannabinoids.[9]

I tell patients that some combination of the body's own opioid and cannabis system will make them feel amazing after exercise, and most people have had this experience. The trouble is, you need to get out onto the trails, the roads, and even the treadmills to experience the runner's high. People with depression — the very people who would benefit most from exercise — often lack the motivation to exercise.

Depression is one of the most common problems I see in my clinic. Depression affects over one hundred million people globally. It is a leading cause of disability in the world. Almost every day someone comes to the clinic complaining of symptoms of depression or anxiety so severe that the symptoms are interfering with their ability to live a normal life. Their function is so impaired that they can't work or manage relationships or attend school.

Declining physical activity and less contact with nature may be contributing to worsening mental health conditions such as depression and anxiety. A systematic review in 2016 found strong evidence linking sedentary screen time with depressive symptoms among adolescents.[10] I talk to my patients about the benefits of physical activity for their mood, and the evidence is strong. In the first place, exercise seems to prevent depression. In 2016 a major review, which included over one million people, looked at numerous studies of the effects of exercise on mood.[11] The study divided participants into groups with low, medium, and high cardiorespiratory fitness. They found that the least active group was 76 percent more likely to develop depression than the most active group, while the medium activity group was 23 percent more likely to develop depression than the most active group.[12]

Exercise not only helps to prevent depression and anxiety, it also helps to treat these common conditions. A randomized trial showed that higher exercise energy expenditure resulted in greater improvement in measures of both physical and psychological quality of life.[13] Large reviews of the medical evidence suggest that exercise is as effective as antidepressants in treating depression.[14] Guidelines in New Zealand and Australia recommend lifestyle interventions such as exercise, improving sleep, and addressing substance use as the first step in treating depression. They suggest using counselling and medications only if patients don't improve with lifestyle interventions. Proponents of exercise as a treatment for depression and anxiety point out that the side effects include huge benefits to the body, which other treatments don't have, and that it is a very cheap treatment. There is also something empowering about taking control of your symptoms by exercising, while some patients may feel disempowered by having to rely on medication. The fact that Big Pharma has nothing to gain is likely a big reason there is less awareness about the benefits of exercise and other lifestyle interventions for mental health conditions.

I tell patients with anxiety, in particular, to go out and exercise every day until they sweat. Indeed, the evidence supports exercising at a moderate intensity for as little as thirty minutes a day. Who can't relate to the need to get out and go on a walk when struggling with stress and anxiety? As an undergraduate in Montreal, although I hadn't yet rediscovered running, I used to walk around my neighbourhood late into the night, working off my nervous energy before returning home to continue studying for a biology exam or complete a set of physics problems.

While exams are, for the most part, a thing of the past for me, stress is a natural product of everyday life. These days my clinics are busy. We see anyone who walks in with an urgent issue. That is the thrill of medicine. To feel that people will turn to you at times of strife was part of why I studied medicine in the first place. On the other hand, there are only so many minutes in a day. Clinics can become congested, weighed down with sickness and need, stuffed with forms and prescription renewals. The sympathetic nervous system is activated, and the stress hormones begin to flow. As stress increases, the mind becomes cluttered, slowed, distractible. Running is the best medicine for this state of affairs.

When I run between clinics, which I try to do almost every day, I feel as if I've taken a Valium. This is ironic because I've never taken a Valium. Despite never having had a benzodiazepine in my life, I have heard so many patients with anxiety and withdrawal symptoms request more and more benzodiazepines and describe the immediate and positive effects of this group of medication. They feel calm, they forget about their stress, they relax, their heart rate and breathing slows, they feel, in short, amazing. That is exactly how I feel after running. I feel amazing, and unlike with benzodiazepines, which quickly lose their effect after regular usage, the positive mental and physical effects of running only strengthen with time as the brain becomes primed to expect to feel amazing, as it associates running shoes, physical exertion, and sweating with that happy post-run euphoria. And also, unlike the euphoria associated with drugs, running does not impair your judgment; it just makes you feel good.

My afternoon clinics are, if anything, crazier and more unpredictable than my morning clinics, and I sit there in my post-run euphoria as if in the eye of the storm. Chaos and strife swirl around me, but I remain calm. People ask Murakami what he thinks about when he runs. He says he doesn't think about anything. "I just run. I run in a void. Or maybe I should put it the other way: I run in order to acquire a void." Murakami's "void" is another term for the calm, the quiescence that we feel after we run. Gretchen Reynolds calls this the "Buddha Brain." She describes a study where men were shown a slide show designed to drive them into a rage. If they had exercised, on a subsequent viewing they were less piqued. She quotes the author, advising, "[I]f you know you're going to be entering into a situation that is likely to make you angry, go for a run first."[15]

Jonathan Beverly, a writer, editor, and accomplished runner, wrote an article called "The Lovely Loneliness of the Solitary Run" that resonated with me. To Beverly, solitary running is a haven, a place where he can contemplate natural beauty or explore "the myriad trails of ideas within my head. The two often come together, with a patch of nature providing the solitude and the loneliness creating the mind-set with which to notice and enjoy it."

Running was rediscovered by millions in the dark spring of 2020 when lockdowns were first imposed across much of the world. Gyms were out, but exercise was in. Plenty of people ate more comfort food and gained weight, but many others like me ate more comfort food and exercised more, so the two kind of cancelled each other out. Although there were no real live group races to train for, I found myself running more, and more consistently than ever before. Running became the easiest, safest, healthiest, and best escape from the pandemic. Within our six-foot bubbles, we moved gingerly along paths and sidewalks, weaving and turning our heads, holding our breath, wearing our masks, trying to coexist and survive. We needed to quiet the clamouring voices of crisis and despair. It was the anandamide, the calm, the void, that we were after.

The pandemic also pushed my family and I closer to nature than ever before. My wife, instead of finding a new museum or exhibit to discover, found us new parks, new trails, new rivers, new cycle paths, more nature, more fresh air, more swimming, more walking — we couldn't get enough. And we were not alone. Nature has never been so prized and, in Canada at least, so crowded. One day in August we were turned away from an entire forest because capacity had been reached. This was a brave new world. My kids got stronger and stronger as the days turned into weeks and the weeks into months. The lockdown became a siege, with humanity on the inside and the virus all around us. But every time we got outside and exercised, we were momentarily released from our imprisonment.

New exercise habits spread like a plague of wellness. Cycling was also ascendant, and stationary bicycles, such as the Peloton, became more and more popular. My wife began to use one, exercising with increasing passion and intensity. My colleagues and I, when we did go to the office, would show up in increasingly casual "active leisure wear." Most of the time we were on the phone, so we didn't need to dress to impress quite as much. The pandemic changed so much about life — jobs, school, schedules, commuting, the boundaries between work and home. We shopped online for new workout outfits, new shoes, new gear. My dad scoured his neighbourhood in Maryland trying to buy a set of weights before finally giving up.

The world was in a terrible state; people were suffering, but things were also better, and many people were somehow thriving. We were discovering previously untapped stores of resilience, finding different and perhaps better ways to organize our lives, to be with our families, to work, to move, to live. Change was accelerated and the catalyst was a virus. Amid all this change and uncertainty, some lucky people had the reassurance of being in nature, of being free to run. Many fled the cities, but many others remained locked into urban settings with too little access to nature, too few safe places in which to move. Some cities closed streets in an effort to give people more space, but whether this will lead to long-term shifts in urban planning remains to be seen.

One weekend I woke up at 4:00 a.m., full of energy. I crept downstairs trying not to wake my family, still peaceful in their beds. I began to listen to the radio, and before long was entranced by a fascinating

Italian-English accent that belonged to an addiction psychiatrist named Henrietta Bowden-Jones. She grew up in Milan then moved to England for her schooling. She said she came to the field of addictions because of a fascination with the mind and the experiences of seeing young men and women injecting heroin in the parks of Milan flanking her walk to school in the 1970s. Many others would have witnessed the same events and experienced only disgust and revulsion, but not Henrietta. In the interview she described becoming interested in behavioural addictions and gambling addiction in particular. The interviewer asked her how she coped with the emotional trauma of her work, and her answer left me ringing with understanding — "Running." She described running an hour at a time to shed the stress of her work.

It's often much easier to think and plan when running. I have all my best ideas and come up with my most ambitious plans when running. When do other people do their best thinking? I remember reading that Alan Turing, who developed some of the fundamental ideas behind computing, artificial intelligence, and cryptography, began to run while at Cambridge and had moments of inspiration while on the fields running between Cambridge and the nearby cathedral town of Ely. One summer day in 1936 he was so overwhelmed by ideas during a run that he lay down in an apple orchard to focus on his thoughts. He ran the fifty-kilometre route to Ely and back frequently. He used running to cope with the stress of his work, saying that the only way he could release the stress was by running hard. He was so fast he even tried out for the British Olympic Team, but an injury kept him off the team.

Exercise reduces anxiety, at least in part, by causing the neurons that release the calming neurotransmitter gamma-aminobutyric acid (GABA) to proliferate. GABA inhibits excitatory brain activity, thus releasing more GABA makes a person feel calmer. The brains of animals that are made to run more go on to develop more excitable neurons and more GABA-releasing neurons. Running also makes you feel sharper and more alert. Though exercise leads to more excitatory neurons and synapses, animal studies suggest GABA-releasing neurons are also more likely to be activated in response to stress. In one study, mice who ran on wheels regularly recovered from the stress of being placed in cold water more quickly than sedentary mice.[16]

Exercise boosts our mood and cognitive function through the production of brain-derived neurotrophic factor (BDNF). The trigger to release BDNF after exercise may be anandamide, the body's endocannabinoid molecule, which is itself released by exercise and may be responsible for the runner's high.[17] Thus, it should be no surprise that running, in particular, boosts the production of BDNF. Running leads to a healthier body, and BDNF helps ensure that running also leads to a healthier brain. BDNF promotes the growth of dendrites, the long arms connecting neurons to each other. It strengthens synapses — the bridges between neurons. And finally, BDNF makes stem cells turn into healthy new neurons.[18]

More and more evidence shows that endurance exercise actually stimulates the growth of new brain cells and is linked with improved cognitive function.[19] Most exercise-induced brain growth in humans occurs in the hippocampus. Exercise is also neuroprotective — it improves factors related to neurodegenerative diseases such as age of onset, progression, and severity of symptoms. Finally, exercise improves recovery from a range of injuries to the brain.[20]

Exercise makes young people smarter and is associated with better school performance. A study of a million young Swedish men who joined the military found that markers of physical fitness were correlated with higher IQ. This correlation was true even among identical twins, showing the importance of physical activity during childhood. The boys with higher IQs also went on to have higher paying careers.[21] Other studies show that after only six weeks of regular exercise individuals have improved working memory and visuospatial processing.[22] Regular exercisers also improve their performance on creative problem-solving tests after a short workout.[23]

Researchers have proposed other explanations for the positive effects of exercise on the brain apart from its stimulation of the release of BDNF. One is that exercise increases blood and oxygen consumption in the brain. Another is that exercise increases neurotransmitter quantity and quality, especially the neurotransmitters that we know impact our mood and cognitive abilities: dopamine, norepinephrine, and serotonin.[24] For example, when we have looked at the genetic activity in the hippocampus of mice that have been encouraged to exercise, it looks similar to those of other mice that were given serotonin-boosting medications. Thus, exercise may work in part by boosting serotonin levels, the same effect of most common antidepressants, such as Prozac.[25]

Dopamine is the brain's principal molecule of pleasure. The reason we lose the will to be active as we age remains a mystery. My son bounces off the walls, but an elderly person is content to sit quietly for hours. What is different in their brains? A fascinating study that looked at non-human animals noted that this age-related decline in activity is seen across many other species.[26] The author decided that the explanation involved dopamine. Both reduced dopamine release and loss of dopamine receptors seem to contribute to the decline in activity seen with aging. What's more, when dopamine levels are enhanced in the brain of older animals, their activity levels go up. In a real sense, dopamine seems to motivate us to be active. This desire to exercise, in turn, alters our brain's neurochemistry and creates a feedback loop whereby our pleasure molecule drives us to achieve more happiness.

Carl came to see me recently with pain in his right foot that came on predominantly when he was running. I remember Carl telling me on a previous visit that he trained for races up to the half-marathon distance. On reviewing his chart, I noted that the month before Carl had been seen by his psychiatrist for severe depression. He told me that his mood had worsened as his foot pain interfered with his training, and this made it harder for him to control his mood symptoms.

Carl had first started running on the advice of his psychiatrist. This was promoted for a time through a running program called "Run With It" based out of Ottawa's mental health hospital. The program was started by a woman named Peggy Hickman after she discovered how helpful running was for controlling her schizophrenia symptoms. Peggy said in an interview that when her psychiatrist first suggested she try running at the age of fifty-eight, she thought he was "off his rocker" but decided to give it a try.

For patients such as Peggy and Carl, managing running-related injuries becomes even more important than it is for the average recreational runner because exercise is their medicine. I examined Carl, and after hearing his description that his heel pain was worse first thing in the morning and then stressing his plantar fascia to elicit tenderness, I told him he probably had plantar fasciitis, and we reviewed the stretches and exercises that would help speed his recovery.

Angela told me during our first visit that she had such bad anxiety during high school that she would miss school for days and even weeks at a time. A child psychiatrist diagnosed her with generalized anxiety disorder in grade ten. She began to see a counsellor for cognitive behavioural therapy, a powerful type of treatment that works to retrain the brain's response to stress-inducing situations. Her psychiatrist also started her on citalopram, a serotonin-boosting medicine that treats patients with anxiety and depression.

Grade ten was tough for Angela, but she got her symptoms under better control over the next year. In grade eleven, she joined the cross-country team and discovered the effect running had on her mood. "In the morning at school, I would feel so wound up and tense, then after practice I'd try to remember why I had felt that way, but I couldn't. All my anxiety was gone."

She raced with her high school and even travelled to provincial races. Her grades got better, and she felt comfortable with herself in social settings.

When I met her, she was in her first year of her undergraduate degree in psychology. She had stopped running for the past year and been off her citalopram for six months. Moving to a new city to start university had been hard on her; she missed her family, her old routines. She tried to exercise but was less motivated, and she felt overwhelmed by her workload.

"My anxiety is the worst it's been in years," she confessed. She had a panic attack before a midterm exam. She found it harder to go out to social occasions and was isolating herself. She complained of poor sleep, headaches, difficulty relaxing, and pain in her neck and shoulders.

As I listened to Angela describe her suffering, I heard echoes of the stories that so many similar patients have shared with me across the years. Anxiety is so common; about 10 percent of people suffer with generalized anxiety disorder during their lifetime. It is a normal and healthy reaction, one that served early humans well. Now, however, it can get out of control. It leads to suffering in part because of pathways in the brain, but also because of the way our bodies are used. Angela had been trapped by sedentary work in class and the library. She was emotionally exhausted, so she thought she was also physically exhausted. I asked her about trying to get back to running. I reminded her how good it made her feel. We agreed to try a variety of treatments. She would reconnect with her counsellor; she would cut out caffeine; and she would make an effort to get outside and be active every day. If she was still suffering, I told her we could restart the citalopram.

Sometimes patients come back after a few weeks, frustrated that my advice of exercise has not had any impact on their mood. Fortunately, there is also science for this situation. I tell them that just as an antidepressant takes four to six weeks to have its peak effect, so, too, does exercise. Studies of rats have shown that even three weeks isn't enough time for exercise to salve anxiety, but six weeks is enough.[27] I have seen a similar time lag in my patients. At our six-week follow-up, they have usually started to feel much better.

Exercise changes our brains and therefore our mental health. Running also draws in other runners, opening the door to forming adult friendships, even at a time in life when many people think the time for making new friends has passed. New friends help you weave a nest of well-being around your life. Children make new friends in the playground. Running can be a passport back to that child-like fellowship. When we feel good around people, we associate them with that good feeling. *That person makes me feel good about myself*, we think. That is the key to friendship.

When a new couple and their young son moved in across the street, I quickly discovered that not only was Jorg, the tall German father, a runner, but he was also fresh from running his first marathon a few months before.

"We should go running together" was the easiest thing to say when I first met him a few weeks later, and then it was simple to text him one morning to arrange a lunchtime run for later that day. As we traced my familiar route around Dow's Lake, I showed him the features of the route, like a child showing a friend the toys in his bedroom: this is where we cross the canal; this is the little peninsula that takes us into the lake; this is where we cross Bronson Bridge back into the neighbourhood.

Afterward, we sat on the front porch, drinking cold water, talking about our families and the renovation work Jorg was doing on his new house.

A few weeks later, after the kids were in bed, we drove to Pine Grove Forest. We parked in a small lot next to signs warning of coyotes. We debated bringing headlamps but decided to leave them behind. Then we set off on the dirt trail.

We ran side by side when the path was wide enough, taking turns leading single file when it narrowed. We came across only a handful of other people out walking their dogs in the late summer light. The ice and snow had been late to melt this year; the rains were relentless, but on this night the ground was dry and the sky was clear. Jorg had found a job as an architect working on a visitor centre for Canada's Parliament, so we talked about how we would fit our runs into our work and family schedule. At one point we lost the path and had to run parallel with a road before we found the path again and continued across the road into a part of the forest that had neat rows of towering pines planted after the original woods had been cut down decades before.

The forest was quiet beyond the sound of our footsteps falling quickly in near unison. In the final moments I imagined we were approaching the finish line of a race. It was still light, but dusk was falling fast. As soon as we stopped to walk the final few metres to the car, we entered a zone of mosquitoes. We talked about how much concern there is about declining insect numbers, and yet it's hard to be concerned when they are biting you on the face. But despite the insects, our new friendship was flourishing, nourished by our time running through the woods and along the canal.

Two weeks later my brother Sascha came to stay, and we went for a morning run that looped up the canal, down the Rideau River, and back home. We set out at quarter to seven on a Sunday morning, but the air was already warm with fresh summer heat. Whatever else was happening in the day or in our lives or in the world, it was so comforting to run together. Earlier that morning, my daughter had vomited on the living room couch after having had stomach pain through much of the night. I had cleaned her up and changed her pyjamas. She probably wouldn't be able to go to school the next day.

But that was a concern for later. Now I was running, now I was rounding the corner and watching as Dow's Lake unfolded before my feet. I was listening to Sascha explain how he was aiming for a step rate, or cadence, of 180 steps a minute, trying to relax his shoulders, trying to find the right zone for his heart rate as he trained for another trail race. Sascha is always learning and improving himself, and I was learning from him. I had followed his lead to become a runner and now I was following him toward drinking oat milk, exploring veganism, and trying to shrink my carbon footprint.

A few months after our Sunday-morning run, Sascha and I ran our first race together. Neither of us had trained as much or as hard as we would have liked. Sascha lamented to me that he hadn't run for three weeks before the race because of his overloaded travel and work schedule.

I was surprised when he told me it would be his second organized race ever, the last being the Warsaw Marathon he had run eight years before, which had, in part, inspired me to become a runner. He told me he didn't need the external motivation; he ran hard and trained consistently without a race. I had started by using races to give me the structure and the goals to push myself, but I also had been in fewer organized races as I matured as a runner.

On a Sunday in early August, we drove thirty minutes to a ski hill to start the 20K trail race. Sascha was excited, in particular, about the trails. He kept saying that this was why he ran, for these trails, for this glorious nature, for days like this. I couldn't have agreed more. There were about two hundred other runners in our event, and our strategy was to start toward the back and speed up as the race progressed. It was a cool morning, and the trails were lovely. Often they were only wide enough for us to go single file, and Sascha paced me, looking back every few minutes to make sure I was keeping up. We knew that the key to trail running was to embrace the descents and just fly down in the spirit of British fell running. The descents were free speed and somehow our feet landed just right. At one point we went down a massive hill that just kept going down a curving gravel trail, and I forced myself to slow down to avoid breaking an ankle or flying forward and breaking a wrist, but Sascha let loose, racing down the trail. *So much for not running in three weeks*, I thought.

We were always either descending or climbing; there were only a few minutes when we were running on a flat, and that felt gloriously easy and straightforward. In the final kilometres we passed more and more runners. I was intoxicated with running, my neurochemicals were surging, the blood was racing through my brain, and I had an epiphany about racing. The other runners weren't part of my race; they were running their own races. Each person was running their own race, set against their body and mind, their training, their goals. Everyone could win this race, even me, despite my relatively casual approach to training in recent months. And when, about fifteen glorious minutes later, we finished, I felt like we had won. I felt so much empathy and so much compassion for other runners. The runner's high transported me to a Buddhist awareness of the oneness of everything.

And the amazing thing is that I felt the same a week later, even after the stiffness had left my calves and I could get out of a chair without making a grunting sound. My body hurt, but my brain had been strengthened by the race. I had bonded with my brother, overcome a challenge, spent two glorious hours in nature, and flooded my body and brain with anandamide, BDNF, and endorphins. This was such a good feeling. Was it too good? Was I addicted to running? Is running addictive or is it the cure for addiction? These were questions I decided I needed to answer.

V RUNNING AND ADDICTION

One day in October, everyone at the clinic was talking about Tara, a twenty-three-year-old woman who had been stabbed to death during the weekend.

"Dr. Ramin, isn't it sad about Tara?" Julie asked as she was leaving the office.

"I knew Tara. Her boyfriend is my buddy; he told me what happened," Brian exclaimed later that day. He went on to explain that Tara was selling drugs, took twenty dollars from a man, and didn't come back with the promised product. Apparently, her boyfriend warned her, "Don't rip him off; he'll kill you." But Tara didn't believe him. Why should she have feared for her life in one of the safest cities on Earth? But the man found her and stabbed her multiple times in the stomach. She was taken to hospital and died the next day.

A life for twenty dollars. Less than the cost of one point of heroin. I listened as people who had known her reflected on the state of the city and the moral universe. In a picture, I saw her dark bangs hanging low over blue-grey eyes. Was she a victim of addiction — her own or that of her killer? Had she lived, would she have been taken by an overdose?

Earlier that week I had received an email from the Ontario Ministry of Health announcing its new opioid addiction and overdose strategy. The strategy was designed to increase access to buprenorphine treatment and naloxone overdose kits. The government was trying to delist high-dose narcotics, trying to get the big doses off the street. It looked like a good strategy, but fewer opioids were coming from prescriptions and more fentanyl powder from China was flooding the streets. A tiny amount of fentanyl could kill many people. How could it be stopped?

The next night I drove to Montreal for the International Society of Addiction Medicine meeting. I looked forward to my runs through the city and along the Lachine Canal. I wanted to hear from my colleagues around the world, listen for solutions to the madness. I didn't want my children coming of age in an epidemic of addiction. We had to fix this; we had to keep pushing for treatments that work, figure out how to prevent people getting started. Maybe a vaccine could be developed. Maybe we as a society have to be more open about addiction.

Earlier that day I had run a slow seven kilometres, punctuated by ten one-minute sprints. I pushed myself hard through the last two sprints, telling myself that this was the hard work that would make me faster, this is where it counted. I woke up in Montreal and left my hotel, running a familiar route to Victoria Square, down McGill Street, and along the Lachine Canal. It was just after six and the sun was still below the horizon. I wore running gloves, but the air was warm. My legs felt stiff from my sprints the day before. I followed the asphalt path until I got to the canal, then switched to the loose gravel trail. One man, who looked to be in his early fifties, passed me going the other direction. His face was a mask of pain, the sweat pouring down. He was pushing himself hard. I was reminded of a moment recently when I had passed a runner while breathing hard, and he looked over at me with a thumbs-up.

"Go for it, have a great run," he urged me.

"You, too" was all I could muster over my surprise.

In my post-run euphoria, the addiction meeting entranced me. Nora Volkow spoke about her priorities in treating and preventing addiction. She is a fascinating woman, having ascended from her medical training in Mexico to become the director of the National Institute on Drug Abuse in the United States since 2002. I was fascinated to learn that she is Leon Trotsky's great-granddaughter and grew up in the house in Mexico City, where he was murdered in 1940. At the meeting, she talked about the risks of cannabis use in adolescents and the need to keep pushing new and existing treatments for opioid addiction. She has inspired a new generation of addiction physicians and researchers, and I was electrified by her words.

In a video from 2012, Nora Volkow explained why she runs: "I'm a very, very restless person, and thus if I don't run in the morning, I will be jumpy all day long, jumpy and anxious, and running allows me to calm myself down and take things more slowly."

She also reflected on the simple beauty of running. "For me, it's really an extraordinary experience to go running. Some of the most exhilarating moments in a given day for me may be that morning, waking up in the morning and seeing the light changing, that incredible sense of well-being that comes when you're running."[1]

One rainy morning after Tara's death, while I waited for a half-marathon race to start, I noticed the cover of a running magazine that showed a young man with green eyes looking into the camera. The headline on the cover read, "King of Pain: Vanquishing Demons with Lionel Sanders." The headline spoke to the addiction doctor in me, so I flipped to the article and found another picture of him. In this one he was wearing a black hoodie and was silhouetted by a grey sky and barren trees. I read that he had just set a new Ironman world record, coming in at 7:44:29 — beating the previous record by ninety seconds.

According to the article, Sanders is self-coached and trains alone in a room in his house. After dropping out of school, he became addicted to cocaine and struggled with heavy alcohol use. The article quotes him: "I didn't feel comfortable with myself unless I was on some sort of drug or drinking and I went into a real dark place."[2]

His description of that feeling reminded me of many similar comments I had heard from my patients. But things turned around for Sanders. He came so close to suicide that he walked into the garage with a plan in mind, but after reflecting on how his death would impact his family, he walked out of the garage and soon afterward began to change his life and his brain through running. That was in 2009. Over the next five years, he got faster and faster. He took part in triathlons and set that new world record in November 2016. He doesn't go to addiction treatment or support groups. He says he is a lone wolf, and training is his recovery plan. People who know him say his greatest strength as an athlete is his ability to tolerate suffering. He has scarred his brain with drugs, and when the voices are screaming to stop, he can push through the pain.[3]

Catra Corbett used running to heal from a stimulant addiction. In a video she explained that things changed for her after she was arrested for selling methamphetamines. "Sitting in a jail cell made me realize, this is my bottom and I need to stop. And, I had to change my life."

She started to run and found that it made her feel better. From someone who loved to party all night and hated running, she became a runner, an athlete. "I've come so far away from that place.... I could have been in jail but running saved my life, running has saved me and made me a better person."[4]

Catra has taken her running to an extreme place, running one-hundred-mile races once or twice a month. She says that she feels high when she is running alone on trails. "People go to AA or whatever, but I don't. My recovery is out on the trail."[5]

Extreme sports, such as ultrarunning, fulfill a need for some patients who are recovering from substance use disorders. Ultras take runners into a cognitive place they cannot reach in everyday life. One form of ultrarunning is the twenty-four-hour race. It doesn't have a start or finish line; instead, there is usually a loop around which runners go as many times as they can in twenty-four hours. In that one day people experience a lifetime's worth of emotion and pain. By means of the simple act of spending twenty-four hours running around a track, they flood their brains with neurotransmitters and overcome seemingly insurmountable barriers.

Lab rats and mice who are able to run on a wheel in their cage tend to seek cocaine less than those who live in cages whose wheels are locked and who are thus forced to be sedentary. A 2014 review of studies examining the effect of exercise on substance use disorders in humans found that exercise increased the rate of abstinence, reduced withdrawal symptoms, reduced anxiety, and improved mood among study participants.[6]

Exercise can help people quit smoking cigarettes. A study of female participants found that vigorous exercise promotes smoking cessation when combined with a cognitive behavioural program.[7] Exercise helps with cravings, withdrawal symptoms, and staying quit. There is a Running Room store down the street from my house that advertises its "Run to Quit" program. The program teaches participants to run a 5K race while at the same time providing them support to quit smoking. Laurence, who ran the program, told me that the store's program had fourteen participants and that two had successfully quit. He also told me that the Running Room was doubling the locations in Canada at which the program would be offered.

Exercise may play a role in cannabis use as well. In one small study conducted by addiction researchers in Nashville, Tennessee, twelve young men and women with cannabis use disorder were asked to come to the lab for ten thirty-minute sessions on a treadmill.[8] These participants were all very sedentary and were not particularly interested in stopping their cannabis use. They exercised at moderate intensity on the treadmills and were told to go about their normal routine otherwise. During the exercise period, participants said they craved cannabis less: the study found that participants smoked nearly six joints per day before the study, less than three joints per day during the two weeks they were regularly exercising, and around four joints per day after the exercise period was over. This was such a short study, but it hints that there may be a relationship between exercise and cannabis use.

In my own practice I use exercise, preferably outdoor exercise, as one of the tools to help patients recover from addiction and from the profound depression and anxiety that often result from damage to the brain following years of substance abuse. It is strange to talk about the "runner's high" with patients who are trying to get through life without feeling the "high" of their drug of choice. I try to explain that a natural high — such as from exercise, love, or a feeling of accomplishment — results in a small release of dopamine and other neurotransmitters. Because this increase is within the brain's capacity to cope, it can be experienced over and over again, and it doesn't result in negative changes in the brain. Using cocaine, however, leads to an astronomical release of dopamine and results in a total depletion of the brain's supply and a significantly decreased sensitivity to further normal influxes of dopamine. Using addictive substances causes such an imbalance in the brain that after a brief and intense high, the brain is less responsive to normal pleasure.

In fact, when coming off cocaine, cocaine users go through a "crash" that leaves them feeling depressed, tired, and completely without motivation. That is why people who have used drugs for long periods of time begin to need drugs to feel "normal." At all other times, they are in a withdrawal state in which they feel much worse than they did before they began using drugs. That is also why people with addictions are less motivated by the same everyday drives as other people, such as nurturing their relationships or taking care of their health. When the brain is less responsive to dopamine, a person's motivation to be active declines. Addiction produces such a state.

Scott Douglas, an editor at *Runner's World* and author of numerous bestselling books about running, wrote a remarkable book about the mental health impact of the sport entitled *Running Is My Therapy*. In the book, Douglas speaks to a therapist named Frank Brooks, who believes many patients who use substances are self-medicating for anxiety or depression. "They're trying to alter their mood. One of these reasons why it's so difficult to maintain sobriety over time is not because people don't have good intentions or don't know what to do, it's that they become overwhelmed by the anxiety or they slip into a depression, and self-medicate again," Brooks says.

This is a theme I have heard again and again. A period of sobriety smashed by an unexpected stressor, such as a big fight with a friend or partner, a setback at work, being reminded of an abusive relationship, a health scare, so many things. The solution here is not to avoid stressors — every life is filled with a steady stream of entropy, bad news, and bad luck — rather, it is to develop healthy coping strategies. We all want to change how we feel at times: some people use drugs; some people, exercise; and some people do both.

Scott Douglas admits in *Running Is My Therapy* that he struggled with alcoholism and depression himself:

> As things continued to deteriorate, I began drinking secretly. I'd stash easily hidden easily chugged 50-ml bottles of vodka in the attic or my clothes chest. When my wife realized this was happening, I hid liquor outside the house, often in spots I'd stop at in the last mile of a run. I was disgusted with myself, not just for how much time and mental energy I spent thinking about drinking, but even more so for regularly lying to and disappointing my wife.

After seeing a counsellor for cognitive behaviour therapy, Douglas tried to return to social drinking. During this period he struggled with constant doubts about whether he should drink today, whether he could have a second beer or another glass of wine. In the end he decided to stop drinking completely. At first, his mood was even worse. He had lost the rewards of alcohol, so he increased the intensity of his running. He ran more with friends until, after a few months, he stopped thinking about alcohol.

A remarkable case report further showed me the power of exercise to treat alcohol use disorder.[9] In the report two researchers from Germany tell the story of Mr. A, a thirty-seven-year-old man from the former Soviet Union who was then living in Germany. He was divorced, had two children, and was unemployed. He grew up in the Soviet Union, and his father died of alcohol cirrhosis. Mr. A left school at age fifteen, which is also when he began drinking homemade alcohol. He began to drink more heavily and spent two years in prison (for unspecified reasons). He began to smoke while in prison. In 1997 Mr. A moved to Germany with his wife. He worked in construction and, over several years, began drinking at work, as much as two bottles of vodka a day. In 2010 his wife divorced him. He continued to drink heavily, to the point that he developed alcoholic cirrhosis, which led to acute liver failure, pancreatitis, encephalopathy (inflammation and damage to the brain), diabetes, and an infection of the blood called sepsis.

For a time in 2011 he was so sick that he lived in a nursing home. He recovered to the extent that he could get access to alcohol, which he did, leading to another relapse. At this point he was admitted to a long-term addiction facility because of suicidal thoughts and encephalopathy. At the time of his admission Mr. A was in very bad shape. He had been bedridden and only recently started to walk again with the help of physiotherapy. He had a history of obesity but had lost thirty-five kilograms due to his severe illness. His physical exam revealed total muscle atrophy, abnormal gait, and reduced shoulder movement due to a tendon injury resulting from an alcohol-related fall. Mr. A complained of chronic severe pain in his lower back and left shoulder, and numbness and tingling in his legs resulting from nerve damage from alcohol toxicity.

When his treating physicians suggested a combination of work, sport, and drug treatment, Mr. A was pretty skeptical. Sport therapy? He had last been physically active during his childhood. But his condition was so bad that he agreed to try anything. His therapists designed an exercise program, and his exercise therapy began in groups of six to ten other patients, with some individual therapy. Initially, Mr. A struggled. His chronic pain, cravings for alcohol, depression, and insomnia impaired his ability to participate, but he persevered. After only four weeks he began to show good progress. His weekly alcohol breath tests were all negative. Within three months his training program was intensified, and he started to do longer and more demanding workouts.

Soon Mr. A became one of the strongest and most involved participants in the program. He was noted to be more self-confident, and he communicated about his feelings. He had transformed into a social and helpful member of the group. Within a year he felt strong enough to go on a week-long biking trip. Group biking in nature became one of his hobbies. He spoke about the effects of exercise on his emotional well-being, explaining that exercise helped him cope with feelings of loneliness and boredom and made him feel good. His mood and sleep improved; his back and shoulder pain lessened. His cravings for alcohol continued to wane. After three years of this program, Mr. A had not relapsed to alcohol. He lived independently in an apartment and worked four days a week for a construction company.

What accounts for this remarkable transformation? Mr. A himself says exercise was a key factor in his recovery, and the authors feel the evidence supports this view. They remind us there is evidence that exercise improves both mental health conditions and substance use conditions, such as alcoholism. Of course, this is the story of only one man's journey and may not be representative. But a review in 2016 concluded that there is evidence that exercise is a useful tool to treat alcohol use disorders. The authors postulate that exercise may impact the areas of the brain involved in addiction. A key challenge in this situation, as Mr. A demonstrated, is motivating patients to participate in physical activity both at the outset of treatment, and in the long term. We also need better evidence for the right duration, intensity, and frequency of exercise to treat this condition.

One afternoon I was seeing Joshua, a fifty-two-year-old former tennis coach who had developed an opioid addiction after a terrible car accident. Like many of my patients, he first felt the powerful calming and soothing touch of opioids while hospitalized for the trauma. He was prescribed OxyContin pills, then fentanyl patches, and for a time he was able to get back to rebuilding his life and rehabilitating his body. But soon the opioids didn't give him the same comfort as in the past, and he sought out new sources — buying stronger fentanyl patches on the street and looking for new ways to deliver the opioids to his brain by smoking his medication.

This went on for a time before he came to treatment. When I met him, he was struggling with the terrible symptoms of opioid withdrawal. Going through opioid withdrawal is like having a terrible flu. Every organ that is impacted by opioids goes into full revolt. A patient begins to feel sweats, then muscle aches, then nausea, vomiting, worsening abdominal pain, rising anxiety, and finally a crescendo of pain. I assessed Joshua's withdrawal and administered 2 mg of buprenorphine. Within an hour his symptoms had improved by about half. I gave another 2 mg, and after a few more hours, his sweating had stopped and the pained look had left his face.

These days his pain is very well controlled on 6 mg of buprenorphine, which he takes as a pill once daily, and he is able to once again get on with his life. He told me he loved tennis and had an amazing career, training some top players in Canada. "But do you know what gave me the biggest rush ever?" he asked. I thought of his days abusing opioids and of his career, but he surprised me. "Finishing a marathon," he said. He told me he had finished ten marathons and nothing else came close to the euphoria and personal satisfaction of reaching the end of those 26.2 miles.

When I last saw Joshua, he told me that since he had stopped using fentanyl patches, he was back to playing tennis and had begun to run up to an hour almost every day. He said he didn't go fast — he wasn't training for any races — he just needed to run. "If I didn't run, I'd go crazy," he told me. He still had some pain in his knees and back, but the running helped keep it under control. On the days he didn't run, he swam for up to ninety minutes, which also helped soothe his back discomfort. For a time his life had been controlled by his cravings for opioids; now he craved exercise. I encouraged him to not overdo it, to rest if he felt the need. He smiled and reassured me, "I haven't felt this good in years."

Exercise has become an important way my patients with substance use disorders cope with stress. I had been following Julie, another patient with an opioid addiction, for just over one year when she was diagnosed with breast cancer. The first day I met her, she told me that she was being followed at the breast clinic for a lump that had been found a few months earlier. At each visit I would ask her for an update. She missed a few appointments but eventually went for the biopsy they had ordered. Then she got the results. "I knew something was wrong. Everyone was treating me really nicely and talking in quiet voices, then they told me it was cancer," she said through her tears.

Since I had known her, Julie had gone from sniffing heroin almost every day to living a drug-free life. At my encouragement she had applied for a subsidized gym pass and started going to the gym four or five times a week. It was her anxiety and painful memories that had led to her heroin use. She used opioids to numb her feelings. Now she had to cope with the emotions of her cancer diagnosis. "It's giving me cravings. I've started having using dreams again," she told me. What's more, she had lost her gym subsidy, hadn't been able to afford the membership for a month, and had stopped exercising. She began to have panic attacks.

It was only months later, when she had been through successful treatment for her cancer and started to exercise again, that she began to get back to a better place. Six months later she returned for a follow-up. She looked calmer. She told me she wasn't having cravings for heroin any longer and had started taking her dog for long walks every evening.

What if we could have prevented Julie's addiction in the first place? The evidence linking sports and exercise with preventing teen substance use is a quagmire. It's hard to compare playing on a college football or soccer team, and all the concomitant baggage that comes along with such sports, to cross-country training or gymnastics. But there are a few intriguing pieces of knowledge we can uncover. First, sport participation among youth actually *increases* alcohol use on average. This may be because of bonding rituals and social scene associated with many high school and college team sports. On the other hand, tobacco and illicit drug use among adolescents is clearly *decreased* when they participate in sports.

What happened in Iceland in the last twenty years really opened my eyes to the potential for physical activity and good parenting strategies to prevent substance use. In the 1990s Iceland had a serious problem with substance abuse among teens. It had the highest rate of teen drinking in Europe, and it also had a high rate of teen marijuana use and smoking initiation. A number of health and addiction researchers promoted the idea of letting teens get high on the euphoria of exercise and self-expression rather than on illicit drugs. They looked at surveys showing the difference between teens who had problematic substance use and those who didn't and found a few important protective factors. The kids without problems were more likely to be involved in organized sports three to four times per week, spent more time with their parents, felt cared about at school, and were not out late in the evenings. Using this information, a lot was done to educate parents around the importance of physical activity for kids and the importance of spending quality time with their kids.

The government made physical activity for youth easier and cheaper to access. It created subsidies and promoted joining teams. You don't find Icelandic teens loitering around after school anymore; they are nearly all doing something active or something creative. Interestingly, a curfew for teens was also put into place. So instead of hanging out and looking for trouble, teens are either playing sports or are home with their families. The results were incredible. The percentage of fifteen- to sixteen-year-olds who had been drunk in the previous month fell from 42 percent in 1998 to 5 percent in 2016. The percentage who had ever used cannabis fell from 17 to 7 percent, and those smoking cigarettes every day fell from 23 to 3 percent.

In 2015 Mike Ferullo, a social worker who was then in his late sixties, founded the Boston Bulldogs, a running club for people in recovery or affected by addiction. Ferullo struggled with an addiction to heroin as a young man before getting sober, taking up running seriously, and going back to study social work. He had a vision of using running as a tool for people to achieve sobriety. Through the Boston Bulldogs, he provides such a tool, connecting people in recovery with running buddies, coaches, a regular running group, and other supports.

Ferullo's efforts in Boston, employing exercise to combat Big Tobacco, Big Alcohol, Big Cannabis, and the opioid epidemic, can seem almost laughable. But time and again the scientific evidence and the experience of a country like Iceland supports the notion of exercise as a way to make people feel happy, healthy, and calm. Through exercise we achieve new highs.

VI RUNNING FASTER

On race day I awoke to a dark sky and the sound of rain. The water was streaming down the windows and dripping into the garden. The day before, I had received a message confirming that while the race was still on, the course would be adjusted because of flooding on the trails. The forecast was for constant rain and temperatures a few degrees above freezing. I planned to run without a hat or gloves as I expected that once they became waterlogged, they would just slow me down. With a banana and a mug of tea at my side, I drove the thirty minutes through Gatineau to the starting area at the base of a ski hill. The earth was overflowing with water. Each time the rain broke for a moment, I knew it was only a temporary reprieve. The rain seemed to fall harder with each renewal. I saw two runners wearing Amsterdam Marathon jackets talking excitedly about their racing strategy. Dozens of children ran in and out of the crowds of tech-clad adults.

The announcer called the runners to the start line for my event, the half-marathon. We stood in the rain as an organizer explained the course changes made because of flooding. Only about eighty of us had made it to the start line. I wondered how many runners, if any, were deterred by the weather. After a few more delays, the starting horn sounded and we were off.

You can run the same path again and again, but it never feels the same. Exactly one year earlier I had crossed the same start line on a sunny morning. This time, I scrambled up the mountain path as rivulets of water ran toward me. I turned left onto a flat patch of gravel before again turning onto a steep descending mud trail. After two kilometres, we climbed past the MacLaren Cemetery.

We skirted the edge of the cemetery and turned down a steep hill. We passed by an old mill, ran under the highway, and found ourselves deep in the Gatineau forest. Most runners stuck to the edge of the trail to avoid the deeper pools in the middle. I ran alongside a few runners, and we got into the easy conversations forged by our shared adversity, bonded by the challenge we had set ourselves. At the halfway point, I passed through a covered bridge, ran a few hundred metres on the road and turned around. I caught up with a tall, lean runner in his early fifties. He told me his name was Luke and he had been racing since his twenties. Wearing shorts and a T-shirt, he admitted to feeling the cold. As our feet struggled to find patches of solid ground, Luke lost his footing and came down hard. Well over six feet tall, he plummeted into the water with a great splash. I looked him over quickly and saw some blood on his leg, but he said he felt okay and we kept going at the same pace.

As the course neared its end, we once again climbed the hill toward the MacLaren Cemetery. Each step up the hill was a challenge, but I felt fresh in the cold morning. I was not wearing a watch that day, so I had no idea if I was on pace. The last three kilometres were mostly downhill. I had learned in the last year to embrace speed on the downhills, and I felt myself letting go as I sprinted toward the finish. Race officials guided me toward the final chute. A man's voice announced each finisher over a loudspeaker. I felt like there was a runner right behind me, but when

I turned around, no one was there. I crossed the finish line. Some of the runners I befriended during the race came up to high-five me. Luke came in just over a minute behind me. I drank water and ate two orange slices and a banana.

Everything was wet. I changed into a dry shirt, took off my mud-caked shoes and got ready for the drive home. A few minutes later, I started to feel the runner's high overcome me. In the background, I had very loud classical music on the radio. And then I yelled with joy. "Yeaaaaaaah!" Trying keep my eyes on the highway, looking for errant deer that sometimes venture onto the road, I felt alive. I crossed the bridge over the swollen Ottawa River, which is the border between Quebec and Ontario. I stopped at a light and noticed the Notre-Dame Cathedral beside me. Two large black cars flanked the entrance, and a crowd of people huddled together in the rain. A funeral was ending. An old woman in black was hugging a younger man; a middle-aged woman held a young girl wearing a pink dress. The sky had a majestic sombre quality.

May 6 is a day with special significance in running history. It was on May 6, 1954, that Roger Bannister broke the barrier of the four-minute mile. Decades later on May 6, 2017, the Olympic marathon champion Eliud Kipchoge tried to run down a new barrier — the two-hour marathon. As the star runner at the heart of Nike's Breaking2 program, he and two other runners — headed by a phalanx of pacers and clad in hyper-efficient running shoes — set out at 5:45 in the morning to run 17.5 laps of a specially designed course at the Monza Formula 1 track in Italy.

The day after Breaking2, I met a fellow runner named Leo at a party my wife and I hosted. He told me that he stayed up all night to watch the race. It had been years in the making and cost tens of millions of dollars. And it was a glorious failure. Kipchoge was nearly on pace for so much of the race, but he slowed in the final twenty minutes. He came in at 2 hours and 25 seconds. It was 2 minutes, 32 seconds faster than the world record. But those glorious numbers would not go into the records because Nike hadn't adhered to the rules around pacers, the lead vehicle, and the delivery of drinks to the runners. Leo and I talked about how long we had been anticipating the race, the suspense, the drama, and the greatness of Kipchoge. Three elite racers had started, but only Kipchoge came even close; the next runner was over six minutes behind him.

But it was not the time on the clock that interested me so much as the science behind the project. The running world was electrified by the discoveries and resources that Nike and other groups poured into the program. For a year before Nike's Breaking2, I had followed the news from the competing programs and read about the theories of exercise physiology and engineering that were being endlessly refined to push runners toward the two-hour goal. It was our new four-minute mile. Teams of scientists travelled to Ethiopia and Kenya to work with the runners in their home training regions. Kipchoge trained in Eldoret, the humble marathon-running capital of Kenya. Other runners trained at the Yaya Village outside of Addis Ababa. Every variable was optimized in the buildup to the race: a flat course, the perfect temperature, the perfect running regimen. Nike had to pay Kipchoge one million dollars just to stay in the program and avoid running in the London Marathon, which he had won in 2015 and 2016. After his glorious failure, Kipchoge would go on to win the Berlin Marathon in 2017.

And then two years later, on October 12, 2019, he finally did it. Running through a park in Vienna, again with every variable controlled for, wearing Nike's latest speed-enhancing shoes, cheered on by thousands of fans, Kipchoge ran a marathon in 1 hour, 59 minutes, 40 seconds. When it finally happened, it was news, it was exciting, but it wasn't four-minute-mile exciting. It all had a whiff of anticlimax about it for me. It was an arbitrary goal that one man achieved. Eliud Kipchoge is the fastest marathoner that has ever lived; he is a wonderful runner. But can millions of runners around the world share in his glory? After my initial skepticism I have come to realize that there are lessons we can all take away from this project: lessons about pacing, about footwear, and about grit and perseverance.

The lessons of the sub–two-hour marathon programs have been added to the rich tapestry of training advice that stretches back to Classical Greece. Both Aristotle and Plato offered advice on how to train. In 1782 a *Medicinal Handbook for Runners* was published in Breslau with advice on how to run faster and increase stamina.[1] In the pre-scientific era, idiosyncratic methods were promulgated, adhered to, replaced, and then rediscovered. Many ancient practices are still in use, in part because modern training recognizes that using a variety of approaches is most effective. My handbook was *Runner's World: Complete Guide to Running*. A few months after I started running regularly, I stopped at a bookstore on my way home from work to buy it. As I held the thin volume in my hand, I envisaged how it would transform my running.

Amateur running has been transformed, as witnessed by the fact that people have been running faster than ever in recent years. Comparing contemporary amateur runners from today with the great champions of the past is impressive. To take one example, the winning time of the marathon at the 1936 Olympic Games was matched by the time of the best amateur runner in the 50–55 age group of the 2012 Berlin Marathon.[2]

Over the past fifty years the world has seen the rise of the East African runners. Like the Finland of Nurmi, Ethiopia is an Eden for runners. The first Ethiopian to make his mark was Abebe Bikila. In the Olympic marathon of 1960, the favourite was Sergei Popov, the world record holder from the Soviet Union.[3] But Emperor Haile Selassie had given his blessing to a European who was living in Ethiopia in the 1950s to train a group of Ethiopian runners for the Olympics. They trained in Addis Ababa, eight thousand feet above sea level. Right before the Rome Olympics, Abebe found that his new shoes were giving him pain, so he decided to run barefoot. He and a Moroccan runner led the pack of runners as they made their way through the Italian evening, their path lit by soldiers holding torches in an evocation of the ancient Olympics.[4] Abebe surged past the Moroccan and beat him by twenty-five seconds in a new world record time of 2 hours, 15 minutes, and 16 seconds.

Eight years later, this dominance would be consolidated. At Mexico City's 1968 Olympic Games, athletes from Ethiopia and Kenya dominated most of the races that historically had been won by European runners.[5] Since that time, running has become a sport increasingly dominated by Ethiopians and Kenyans.

The first time I saw elite runners racing in-person was a hundred metres from my home on a cool evening in May 2014. The great Kenyan runner Mary Keitany sprinted by, with a group of other women a few minutes behind. She had been pregnant the year before then come back faster than ever, and she would go on to win the New York City Marathon a few months later. In 2017 she set a world record at the London Marathon.

What's more, the best Kenyan runners seem to come from specific villages. In 1990 only one athlete in the top fifty male marathoners was from Kenya. In 2010 thirty of the top fifty marathoners were Kenyan, and most were from the Kalenjin ethnic group. There are only 3.5 million Kalenjins in Kenya. To try to understand this dominance, researchers have mulled over innumerable variables, including population genetics, food intake, social organization, blood type, maximal oxygen consumption, lactate threshold, running economy, muscle morphology, muscle fibre typing, childhood training, and altitude. Despite this intense study, they have found only partial answers.[6]

The formative effect of walking and running to get to school is a recurrent theme in studies of Ethiopian and Kenyan runners. One study in particular found that Kenyan boys who ran or walked long distances to school had VO_2 max values 30 percent higher than boys who did not have far to go, even if they did not formally train at sports.[7] Two other studies looking at Ethiopia and Kenya also cited childhood endurance activity as a key factor in determining which boys would go on to become great runners.[8]

A tough childhood produces incredibly strong runners. Yannis Pitsiladis observes that the average European child engages in twenty to forty minutes of vigorous physical activity per day compared to 170 minutes for the average Kenyan child. Pitsiladis is an exercise physiologist based in the United Kingdom who worked in Ethiopia trying to find a runner and a training program that could break the two-hour marathon in a competing program to Nike's. In an evocation of a mythical quest, Yannis went to Ethiopia to find the hero. He tested young runners one by one. He believed East Africans dominate road races because, from an early age, running shapes their lives.

When I think of runners training in Iten, the dusty town in the Kenyan highlands that has become synonymous with distance running, I often think of the tall, (sometimes) bearded Englishman Adharanand Finn. Finn wrote a delightful book, *Running with the Kenyans,* in which he recounts the six months of 2011 he spent living and running in Iten. Finn's goal for the trip was to find the secrets of Kenyan running. He spoke with great athletes, visited the high-altitude training centres frequented by runners from around the world, and ran the dusty roads leading out from the city. He posits that the keys to their success include the "tough, active childhood, the barefoot running, the altitude, the diet, the role models, the simple approach to training, the running camps, the focus and dedication, the desire to succeed, to change their lives, the expectation that they can win, the mental toughness, the lack of alternatives, the abundance of trails to train on, the time spent resting, the running to school, the all-pervading running culture, the reverence for running."[9]

I went to meet Finn one weekend in March. To meet him I had to go to Dartmoor, a national park formed from a vast expanse of moorland in the south of England. He hosted a running camp, and I wrote to him asking if I could come and discuss writing with him as well. He was unfailingly gracious and spent time with me talking about his experience writing his running books about Kenya and Japan.

It was my first retreat devoted to running, and it opened my eyes to yet another way to grow as a runner, in a new environment, with a group of talented and dedicated runners, through the gorse bushes of the Dartmoor hills, through darkness and snow. If I had become separated from the others, it would have been so easy to get lost in that featureless wilderness. So I ran close to the rest of the group — a writer, a sports psychologist, a running coach, a computer manager, a farmer, a civil servant husband and wife in their late fifties, and an artist looking for inspiration. I almost lost my way during a night run but found the trail back to our base and left the others to return home just before a major snowstorm hit.

I arrived back in Canada with a new drive to improve, to learn to be a better runner. I had read about these Kenyan running secrets, spoken to Finn and to my fellow runners at the retreat. I knew about core strengthening, protein shakes, hydration and nutrition during runs, weights, the importance of sleep. But how does a runner put these things together to become a better runner? And what is the goal? Is it speed or endurance? Is it to run fast and risk burnout, or to endure late into life? I had met many patients with cautionary tales — intense training, Olympics, cross-country skiing championships — who had developed pain, lost the will to continue their training, and had sometimes given up exercise altogether. I wanted to train for the long term.

The variables an athlete controls in a running program are volume, frequency, and intensity. Roger Bannister and his great Australian rival, John Landy, are a study in two contrasting training programs. Bannister relied on intense interval training because he had to confine much of his training to the lunch hour while a medical student in the 1950s. He saw results, but then he plateaued. It wasn't until he acquired a coach and pacers who pushed him to intensify his training that he was able to break through four minutes.

Landy, on the other hand, intimidated Bannister and all other runners with the intensity and ferocity of his training. Landy had been influenced by witnessing the incredible success of Emil Zátopek, the Czech runner who had won gold medals in the five thousand metre, ten thousand metre, and marathon at the same 1952 Olympics where Bannister had failed to place. Zátopek's training regime was based on the idea that progress arose from subjecting the body to periods of high stress at a fast pace. He believed in training for speed and reducing recovery times between intense periods.[10] Zátopek trained hard.

Landy took up the baton. He would walk to Central Park in Melbourne and run alternating fast and slow laps around the six-hundred-yard gravel track. Five nights a week, after a full day of studying for his agriculture degree, he would run for ninety minutes, pushing himself to his physical limits.[11] He would do longer runs on the other two nights of the week, going more than ten kilometres along the roads leading out of Melbourne. His training method led the victories to pile up. Soon the Australian press saluted his methods. An article from the *Melbourne Herald* taunted its readers: "While you were at the pictures, or square dancing, last Saturday night, John Landy was doing a 10-mile training run."[12]

In the weeks leading up to the 1954 Commonwealth mile championship in Vancouver, Landy would run lap after lap at a blistering pace in view of the public. Bannister, on the other hand, trained in private on a golf course. After each race, including that final one, Landy would hardly appear flushed, while Bannister would collapse and need to recover before he could walk.

There is always a balance between training volume and intensity on the one hand, and the demands of everyday life on the other. I use the Bannister method, insofar as I fit my running into the spare moments between my clinics, teaching, writing, and time with my family. The risk with this method is that it is hard to achieve the volume of miles needed for truly fast results. One of the key factors found to determine race times for novice marathoners is the number of miles run in the month before the race. Running more than sixty miles leads to significantly better results than running forty or fewer miles per week.[13] By contrast, volume is also correlated with overuse injuries and stress fractures.

Most training programs on websites or apps blend gentle runs, interval training, and speed work. And when time is tight or my motivation is low, it is usually the intense workouts that I am more inclined to skip in favour of a gentle 5K jog around the lake. This, of course, does not lead to the best performance.

In fact, "deliberate practice" — training where you have a goal and you work hard to achieve the goal while consciously focusing on form and technique — is a critical part of enhancing performance at almost any activity. A University of Ottawa study found that the best runners were those who incorporated more deliberate practice into their training in the forms of interval training and speed work. What's more, this study showed that the runners rated sessions involving deliberate practice as their most enjoyable.[14] I can definitely relate to this — it's part of the reason racing is so enjoyable — you push yourself even harder and feel the thrill of previously unattained accomplishment.

When I write exercise prescriptions, I explain to my patients that to gauge "moderate" exercise, they should use the talk test. When you are doing aerobic exercise that gets your heart rate near to 80 percent of maximum, you should be able to talk in full sentences, but it shouldn't be easy. The next stage is threshold, where your heart rate is 80–90 percent of its maximum and you can speak a few works at a time. Finally, there is the Zátopek level of anaerobic sprinting, where your heart rate is above 90 percent of maximum and you can only speak in single words. The optimal ratio for these three stages is 70 percent aerobic, 20 percent threshold, and 10 percent anaerobic.[15] Using a heart rate monitor is good, but studies have shown that perceived effort is reliable, and the talk test helps you figure out what zone you are in.

Interval training has been used since Swedish elite trainers developed the concept of *fartlek* (which translates as speed play) in the 1920s. The practice of fartlek is truly playful, as the runner chooses a tree or rock in the distance, sprints toward that goal, slows to a jog, then finds another target to run toward. This was the happy discovery of interval speed training, a critical type of training for any running plan.

Another type of practice is cross-training, which has been one of my favourite topics in running science. There are so many good options. Almost anything you like doing can be considered cross-training for running. Best of all, it is preferable to do a couple of different things. Reviewing the scientific evidence took some of the fun out of cross-training for me as it showed most alternatives to running such as using an elliptical or biking do not improve running performance, but that doesn't mean they aren't enjoyable in and of themselves, and they can still contribute to injury prevention and overall health. The area that is probably most neglected by runners and most beneficial for performance is strength or resistance training.

The exercise prescriptions I provide patients always include two days a week of strength training. I explain that while the lion's share of benefits for health comes from cardiovascular exercise, strength training has a vital and often overlooked role for both health and performance.

Unfortunately, as early as our midthirties, our bodies begin to lose 1–2 percent muscle mass every year for the rest of our lives.[16] *Sarcopenia* is the result, the degenerative loss of skeletal muscle mass and strength. I regularly draw a graph for patients showing their strength and function on one axis and their age on the other. I ask them to imagine things they take for granted now such as climbing stairs or getting out of bed. "If you do nothing to build up or maintain your strength, even those simple activities of daily living will become challenging or impossible after a period of time," I explain in a sombre doctor voice.

I tell them of my realization of this in medical school when I was caring for two seventy-year-old patients admitted to hospital. One cut his own firewood and walked every day and still had impressive visible musculature, while the other had lived a more sedentary life, had no visible muscle mass, and struggled with basic function at home. Although they were the same age, their different lifestyles had resulted in starkly different levels of function.

More muscle also means lower blood sugar and cholesterol. Muscle is the body's central location for burning fat and taking glucose out of the bloodstream. It is also the biggest contributor to the body's resting metabolic rate.[17] I remember our endocrinology instructor telling us that metformin, the first-line diabetes medication we use, "is like exercise in a bottle," insofar as it helps muscles absorb glucose from the blood.

Exercise is better than medication. Having more muscle reduces your risk of developing type 2 diabetes because muscles act as sponges to soak up glucose from the blood and thus reduce the harmful effects of glucose on organs. Strength training causes lean body mass to increase and bad cholesterol levels to fall. Finally, strength training also increases bone strength and increases joint stability.

When Adharanand Finn moved on from Kenya and went to Japan to seek out what the running-obsessed nation of Japan had to teach him, squat toilets and a lack of chairs were two of his key discoveries. The Japanese have the common strengthening exercise known as the squat built into their everyday lives. Exercise physiologists have nominated the squat as the single best exercise because it activates the body's biggest muscles — the gluteal muscles and the large thigh muscles — and it builds power.[18] Finn began to do squats ferociously, but many Japanese people do this exercise as part of their everyday life as they sit on the floor and enjoy the simplicity of squat toilets. In geriatric medicine in the West, we look at a patient's ability to stand up from a regular chair, essentially a very easy form of the squat, as a marker of their functional ability. Getting up from the floor and squatting are far more challenging for anyone who does not regularly practise such activities.

The connection between strength training and performance is not direct. Someone who is extremely muscular will not necessarily be the best sprinter or basketball player. To excel at these activities, you need power, which is the ability to deliver strength in a rapid burst. Power can be developed through practising explosive movement, such as jumping.[19] *Plyometrics* is the term for workouts involving lots of jumping, where the goal is to exert maximum force in short periods of time. A great plyometric workout I enjoy is called "the floor is lava" and involves constantly jumping up, side to side, burpees, and jumping from a squat — all activities that enhance power. One study looking specifically at male distance runners showed that adding a weekly session of plyometrics led to more improvement than standard machine-based strength workouts.[20]

And then there is the core. In medicine, core strength is something it's easy to get excited about, as it's rumoured to prevent lower back pain and maintain function as we age. In running, a strong core is thought to help you maintain good running form as you fatigue during a longer race. The difficulty is agreeing on what we mean by core and how best to make it stronger. The classical image of the core is the rectus abdominis muscles — the elusive six-pack. But the core wraps around the whole body and includes the lower back, the gluteals, and the hip. In fact, hip muscles and deep abdominal muscles have actually been shown to have more impact on core stability and injury prevention than the visible abdominal muscles.[21] Core strength is correlated with athletic performance for running and a variety of other sports.

I remember the joy I felt when I began to regularly incorporate core exercises into my routine. The simple elegance and playful names of the plank, side plank, superman, and bird dog made me feel strong and virtuous. A few times a week, I find myself talking to a patient about the importance of exercise in general and core strength in particular to prevent back pain. I show them a handout with all the important exercises and encourage them to do them regularly at home.

To be really effective, strength training, like endurance training, has to be hard. You can't get better by doing the same gentle run every day, just like you don't get smarter by reading the same book over and over again. You get stronger by obeying what has been called "the one overriding truth in exercise physiology," which is, in a word, *overload*. Overload means you push yourself. You progressively turn up the frequency, intensity, and duration of your training to keep getting new results.[22] Of course, if you turn up the dial too far, you'll end up with an injury or spend all your time exercising, so you need to find a level that is consistent with your exercise and life goals.

A common activity touted to prevent injury and enhance performance is stretching. But science has not been kind to static stretching, which we now believe doesn't prevent injury and probably worsens performance. A review of stretching studies concluded, "Use of stretching as a prevention tool against sports injury has been based on intuition and unsystematic observation rather than scientific evidence."[23] This describes so many of the interventions we have used over the centuries in medicine that have fallen to the discoveries of solid evidence. In fact, stretching before a race may even make you slower. Studies have shown worse performance after stretching, a finding that is thought to be related to lower efficiency of looser muscles or tendons, reduced transmission of force through longer muscle fibres, and the impact of stretching on brain signalling.[24] This effect lasts for about an hour after stretching.

Other types of warm-up aren't harmful, however, and could be part of your pre-race routine. After looking at the evidence around this, I tried the "dynamic stretching" warm-up Alex Hutchinson recommends. You start with a gentle jog, followed by some high-knee running, heel kicks, and walking lunges. The first time I tried this, before a 10K race, another runner came up and said, "It's good to see someone doing a proper warm-up." He had obviously read the same recommendations as me and we bonded over our disdain for static stretching.

The question of what to do after exercise is another matter. You won't be surprised that there isn't much evidence regarding the benefits of stretching or elaborate cool-down routines. In my view, the best cool-down is to just walk — walk to the shower or the kitchen and feel your heart rate slowly coming down and your breathing go back to normal. Stretching after exercise doesn't help prevent the pain and stiffness that you may feel the next day. These pains are known as delayed-onset muscle soreness (DOMS). This term captures in four words an empire of pain resulting from microscopic muscle tears and cellular-level inflammation.

Think of how sore you felt after the most intense exercise of your life. It was bad, but it wasn't that bad, was it? Pain is so much about context. The pain of DOMS is soothed by the knowledge that it results from your body's supreme achievement — running a marathon or completing an intense core-workout class. So it should be less of a disappointment to learn that there's nothing we can do to significantly reduce the intensity or duration of post-exercise DOMS.

For one thing, anti-inflammatories such as ibuprofen and naproxen not only don't help, they probably cause real harm. Lab studies suggest ibuprofen can slow the healing of injuries to muscles, tendons, ligaments, and bones because they block the production of collagen. Since reading this evidence, I have assiduously avoided these painkillers during training and after races, although I believe they do have an important role for other types of pain and illness. Evidence from the Ironman suggests that using anti-inflammatories does not reduce muscle pain after racing. If you look further, you'll find athletes who use these drugs have higher levels of inflammatory markers, kidney impairment, and leakage of bacteria from the colon into the bloodstream.[25]

Sports massage and ice baths seem to have no impact on reducing DOMS either; again, they may worsen the situation. The argument for massage is that it increases blood flow and helps to milk out lactic acid from sore muscles. A Canadian study challenged this belief by showing massage actually clamps down on blood vessels, thus reducing the removal of lactic acid.[26] A randomized trial of the effects of an ice bath after intense exercise suggested they result in more pain and do not diminish the markers of DOMS. Once again, science seems to sweep away time-honoured practices. The simplest way to recover from Zátopek-intensity training or racing is to rest. Insufficient rest can lead to overtraining syndrome and a variety of overuse injuries.

Too much rest, on the other hand, leads to atrophy. It often seems that there are two types of runners — those who train too much and those who train too little. We are told more training is better, and we are also told more rest is better, so it can be hard to find the balance. Too much rest leads to loss of training gains. This process happens as soon as two weeks. That's why it's so common to see a middle-aged man who talks of his glory days as the captain of the high school football team, but who is now sedentary and overweight. Fitness demands continuous attention, tending, and effort. If you do need to take time off to recover from injury, a few short but hard sessions of cross-training can help you maintain fitness for longer.

Along with appropriate doses of rest, appropriate nutrition is also necessary. Before his four-minute-mile race Bannister went to an old friend's house in Oxford and lunched on ham salad, prunes, and custard. This meal is wrong in every way according to modern sports nutrition. I'm not even sure I've ever seen a ham salad. Athletes, like most people, love to talk about food. In particular, athletes want to improve their diets to optimize their performance.

As a physician, I advise patients to eat as much fruit and vegetables as they can get their hands on, and that is the same principle I apply to my own eating habits. We buy mountains of bananas, apples, pears, oranges, berries, and watermelon, but between me, my wife, and my children, we eat so much that we are constantly running out. My philosophy is that if you're eating an apple, you're probably not going to eat something processed and high in fat or sugar.

There is clear evidence that eating processed food is harmful. I often cite a study to families showing how after only two weeks of switching out processed foods (like cookies, granola bars, artificial cereals) for non-processed foods (like bagels, fruits, meat), young people had lower cholesterol, lower blood pressure and lower weight — after only two weeks. There is something uniquely toxic about the liquid sugar made from corn that is stuffed into much processed food, but all "free" sugars have been shown to be harmful. Industry lobbyists have worked hard to promote free sugar. Lobbying prevented the World Health Organization (WHO) from coming out stronger against sugar in the past. At one point the sugar lobby managed to have the U.S. Congress threaten to withdraw funding if the WHO went forward with recommendations to lower sugar consumption. Fortunately, scientific evidence can, over time and sometimes with great effort from public health and advocacy groups, inform policy and change people's minds.

In 2015 the WHO came out with a recommendation to reduce free sugar intake to less than 50 grams per day for adults. The important aspect of this recommendation is it refers to added sugar, not to the sugar found naturally in fruit, vegetables, or milk, none of which have been generally found to be harmful. This is why I give myself and my patients free license to eat fruit. In fact, huge studies from all over the world show that more fruit intake leads to reductions in diabetes, heart disease, and cancer. There is similar evidence with nut intake.

One Christmas I became alarmed at all the sugar on offer in the lunchroom at my clinic, at parties, and in our pantry at home, so I went on a sugar strike. It worked really well for three months. I turned down cookies and cake many times. After a few months my resolve waned, and I allowed myself a little sugar. Before long I was again bingeing on ice cream and chocolate at night after the kids were in bed. This reminded me of the struggles my patients face when trying to abstain from their drugs of choice. Our brains are wired for sugar in a similar manner to the way a cocaine user's brain is wired for cocaine. One problem is that sugar is so much more available than cocaine. The more we treat sugar like a harmful product, restrict its availability, and increase its cost, the more success we will have as a society reducing sugar consumption.

Very active people, however, are able to get away with more carbohydrate and sugar intake than less active individuals. The best recommendations for nutrition were summarized in a position paper by a variety of sports and nutrition groups in 2009. They advise:

1. Consume adequate calories. Fewer than 1,800–2,000 calories per day can lead to reduced muscle mass, bone density, delayed recovery and increased risks of injury, illness and subjective fatigue.
2. Consume adequate carbohydrates. These are important because of the need to maintain blood glucose during exercise and replenish muscle glycogen afterwards.
3. Consume adequate protein. Endurance athletes need about 1.5 g/kg of body weight of protein daily.
4. Healthy fats are needed for energy and should make up about one third of total calorie intake.
5. Stay hydrated. Losing as little as 2 percent of your water content can decrease performance.[27]

Carbohydrate loading with a pasta dinner prior to a race is a wonderful tradition, and there is science to support the basic premise that having more accessible nutrients in your body will improve your endurance. However, this only becomes relevant in exercise lasting longer than about ninety minutes. In longer events such as marathons and ultramarathons most racers top up their carbohydrates as they go along by eating bananas, dried fruit, or sports gels. This greatly reduces the benefits of pre-race loading. Eating during races definitely works as it's been shown that Ironman racers who consume more carbohydrates during races perform better.[28]

Staying hydrated is also important to performance, but water is as good as electrolyte beverages. I was shocked but not surprised when I learned that the companies themselves produced much of the evidence in support of electrolyte drinks, a pattern that cuts across the evidence for many commonly used medications as well.

Post-workout nutrition is another beloved topic of the sporting community. Again, there is science to support the idea that eating after sustained exercise can enhance recovery and training gains. The magic formula is to consume four grams of carbohydrate for every one gram of protein. And this has to be done quickly. There seems to be a window of time post-exercise lasting thirty to forty-five minutes during which muscle cells are very receptive and combining carbohydrates and protein in the 4:1 ratio can help muscles rebuild their glycogen supply by stimulating the body to release insulin.[29]

Numerous studies suggest that milk is a good — and possibly the best — post-workout drink. It has natural sugar, minerals, and protein. Studies have shown that milk leads to better repletion of muscle glycogen stores, less body fat, and better endurance in subsequent workouts compared to so-called sports drinks or even water. Chocolate milk, in particular, has very near the 4:1 carbohydrate to protein ratio that is believed optimal for recovery. This is why for years you couldn't open any runner's magazine without finding a full-page advertisement for chocolate milk.

There is even advice on exactly what to do on race day. My favourite piece of advice in the *Runner's World* manual is about how to cross a finish line: *don't* look at your watch, *don't* slump across the line; *do* look up, put your hands in the air, smile. This simple advice results in a superior finish line photo, but it also makes you feel like a champion when you cross the line, whatever your time.

A more strategic consideration is how to approach hills during a race. An Australian study suggested that most runners make two mistakes when it comes to hills: they go up too quickly and come down too slowly.[30] The problem with trying to maintain a fast pace uphill is that your heart rate increases, and you end up moving toward anaerobic metabolism. You then spend the downhill recovering from this increased effort. You are better off running based on effort; try to keep your heart rate or effort stable. That means you should run (or walk) slowly uphill then speed up a bit downhill and return to your race pace soon after getting back on to level ground.

Pacing is a key factor in a race. Bannister knew that from his physiology research and his own experience on the track. A runner loses more energy by accelerating too early in a race than they save by running slower at another point. Elite runners have an exquisite sense of pace, and the best can run consistently kilometre after kilometre. Finn found this when training with the collegiate runners in Japan as well as with the best Kenyan runners.

A critical element in close races is saving energy for the final kick. In a 1953 race between the Amateur Athletics Association and Oxford University, Bannister made clear his ambition to break the four-minute mile. On the day of the May 2 meet, Bannister drank a mixture of orange juice and glucose, which he had designed to boost performance, then took a twenty-minute warm-up jog. He was paced though the first three laps by his friend Chris Chataway, then in the last lap he unleashed his speed. A journalist described what happened next: "Only the silky-striding Bannister was still in contention; serene and now alone, Bannister sailed on. Wearing the sad, relaxed mask reminiscent of the great Manolete as he delivered the coup de grace in the bull ring."[31] That day Bannister set a new British record by running the mile in 4:03.6. It would take another year to shave off those final seconds.

Bannister had an incredible ability to push his body to the limit and beyond. Contemporaries of his were genuinely concerned that the exertion required for a four-minute mile could be fatal to the ambitious runner. Most amateurs don't push themselves anywhere near their limit; they listen to warnings from their central nervous system to slow down to prevent overheating and muscle exhaustion. A fascinating study from England had cyclists ride as hard as they could over four thousand metres. They were just able to match that time while racing against an avatar of themselves doing the same time on a computer screen. In a clever twist, they were raced against their own avatar set, without their knowledge, to go 2 percent faster than their best time. Again, they were able to match the avatar, showing that our brains can be tricked into pushing to new limits. Thus, the limits of what we are capable of are in part due to physical fitness, but also in large part to the overriding control of our central nervous system.

* * *

A factor that is out of your control is the temperature on race day. Estimates for an optimal temperature for racing range from 3–10°C. The range of 7–10°C was proposed as optimal for Nike's Breaking2 effort in 2017. In fact, the starting temperature for that particular race was 11°C and rose to 12°C over the course of the race. Whether temperature was a factor for the extra twenty-five seconds needed by Eliud Kipchoge to complete the course cannot be known for certain. The Athens Olympic marathon in 2004 had a starting temperature of around 27°C, and the fastest time was 2:10:54. That was a strange marathon, however, as a drunk guy dressed in a kilt ran onto the course and pushed aside the lead runner, who was then passed by the eventual winner, the Italian Stefano Baldini.

One recent spring was unseasonably hot. There was a lot of talk about cancelling race weekend in Ottawa. The Montreal Marathon was cancelled. In the end, the organizers in Ottawa decided to move the start time of the 10K race forward so it started at 7:00 p.m. on the Saturday evening. My daughter and I were watching the race at home. It began to rain only a few minutes after the start of the race; this quickly turned into a thunderstorm. The concerns about heat were alleviated, as the runners were drenched in a summer rain.

The women started first, and we watched as a group of three led the pack — one Kenyan followed closely by two Ethiopian runners. The leader, and eventual winner, was Peres Jepchirchir, who was only twenty-two years old and had a huge lunging stride. As I followed the course of the race, I saw she was about to pass in front of our block, so I grabbed an umbrella and picked up my daughter, and we ran together to the canal to watch. Just as we arrived, we saw Jepchirchir hurtle past with the other two women about thirty seconds behind her. Two minutes later we saw the lead pack of men who were dominated by Simon Cheprot, a Kenyan who was at least a foot taller than the rest of the runners.

We went home to continue watching the race. Jepchirchir extended her lead over the other women and maintained an electric pace until, three metres from the finish line, she stopped. She then slowly took a few steps, crossed the finish line and immediately collapsed. She was lying there when a few moments later the elite men sprinted across, a

Moroccan runner named Mohammed Ziani beating his Ethiopian competitor by 0.4 seconds to claim the prize. Thirty minutes later Jepchirchir was up and speaking to the media about her race. She had pushed herself beyond the limit to win, but her body was so tough that she could recover from such exhaustion in just half an hour.

Because the Olympics were being held later that year, there was a lot of discussion about which runners would meet the qualifying times for their national teams — it was the last day to achieve such a time before final selections were made for the Olympics. Even those who barely made it still wanted the privilege of being selected to travel to the Games so that forevermore they would be known as Olympians. Over two millennia after its start, this remains the highest achievement for any athlete.

The next day I went for my own run. I was one of the only runners out in the humid late afternoon. I kept hoping for some cloud to eclipse the sun, which I felt broiling my skin. I remembered that feeling from our final summer in Cairo in the mid-1990s. The last week before moving to the United Kingdom, I was outside much of the time, saying goodbye to friends, helping organize the move, racing around our neighbourhood. The temperature was over 40°C, and it was like opening an oven. Across two decades, I can still feel it.

I felt the heat as a racer the following year when I entered the 10K during Ottawa Race Weekend. I spent the morning of race day outdoors with my family revelling in the warm sun after several weeks of wet and cold spring days. As I biked to the starting area, I focused on conserving my energy and staying out of the sun. The race was scheduled for 6:30 p.m., and an announcer told us that 10,500 runners were registered.

It was a clear evening and Laurier Avenue was packed with runners bouncing on their heels, readying themselves for the starting horn. A huge Canadian flag was passed over our heads from the elite athletes at the front all the way to the last runners. A friend turned to me and said, "I feel so light; I love this feeling!" The horn sounded and once again I was off racing on familiar roads. Initially, I outran the pacer by a minute or two as I stayed with my friend. We turned left down Elgin Street past hundreds of loud supporters. The course then followed the Rideau Canal where I have logged so many of my training kilometres. For the first four kilometres my body felt fast, and I was enjoying the pace. Then came a slight rise where the course goes up a hill to cross over the canal before coming down the other side. The 5K marker was at the top just before we ran down the ramp and curved back on the other side of the canal.

I passed within one hundred metres of my house, and my family was waiting alongside the path with outstretched hands. It was such a delight to see them, but it was right after that high that I began to tire. Probably I hadn't put in enough training miles, I had slacked off my speed intervals, and the heat! A few hundred metres later, the pacer ran past me with a small group of runners sticking with him. Sweat was pouring into my eyes; my shirt felt like a plastic bag trapping all the heat trying to radiate from my upper body. I desperately wanted to take it off and throw it into the canal, but I decided against this because it was attached to my race bib.

I slowed to a gentler pace and told myself to relax and recover and I would make a final push after the eight-kilometre marker. I continued along the familiar roads, enjoying the crowds and the exhilaration. I wasn't feeling light, but I knew that I would feel amazing once the race was over. At the 8K marker, I increased my cadence, pumping my arms and feeling my breath come faster. The crowds grew as we approached the finish line. One elderly couple held a poster that simply read "Running Encouragement Sign." There was a picture of a man's face enlarged to grotesque proportions with the caption "Smile like this guy."

All of a sudden, I was at the four-hundred-metre marker. The finish line was just around the corner. Every step was an effort, but I remembered everything I had read about the psychological aspects of performance. I remembered the concept that your brain tries to put the brakes on before your body reaches its limit. So I put my arms in the air like a champion as I ran. People all around me yelled like crazy. I felt a wave of emotion; I felt light. I sprinted the last one hundred metres, passing a few racers before stumbling across the finish line. Dozens of runners kept passing the line behind me. I was funnelled forward, given water, my medal, a banana, and half a bagel. I found my friend, and we posed for a photo together holding our medals. It was over.

VII RUNNING HURTS

One afternoon Fenella limped into my clinic. A muscular twenty-four-year-old, she had a cut caked in dried blood over her left eye and a loose and slightly dirty bandage wrapped around her right hand. I looked in her file and saw that at her last visit she had complained of an ankle sprain and possible fracture of her right wrist. I often see people who are assaulted or hurt themselves when they are intoxicated, but Fenella assured me this wasn't the case.

"I run," she told me, pumping her arms back and forth as if sprinting for the finish line.

Running isn't that dangerous, I thought and asked her to explain how she got hurt.

She clarified: "Well, I do parkour."

I was intrigued.

"Tell me about that," I said, using a classic doctor line to get a patient talking.

I had some vague sense of what parkour was, having seen some videos of men racing cars through urban settings. She explained that it is a way of moving, like a martial art, where you jump, slide, or vault around urban obstacles. You run, you run fast, but you intentionally confront objects in your way like walls and overpasses. The movement takes its inspiration from military-style obstacle courses. You jump between buildings, hurtle yourself off bridges. You do flips. Fenella embodied the risky consequences of such a hobby — ankle injury, laceration, possibly a broken wrist.

That night I went home and watched a few more YouTube montages of young men executing high-level parkour. It was impressive, but after a few minutes I realized that the best part of the sport was how fast the guys could run. I couldn't imagine their bodies would last very long taking such a beating. Running can hurt, but our bodies are designed for the repetitive, long haul of running. Parkour is extreme. In this chapter I explore the dangers of more conventional running.

A runner is most likely to be injured if he is male, runs six days per week, and logs more than thirty miles per week. Other factors that increase risk for injury include being overweight or obese and having had a prior injury.[1] It's a truism in medicine that the biggest risk factor for any condition is having had that condition before. A running injury is no exception. Along with patellofemoral syndrome (pain in front of and around the knee) and shin splints, the most common diagnoses to see in runners include Achilles tendon problems, inflammation of the iliotibial band, foot pain due to plantar fasciitis (inflammation of tissue under the foot), and stress fractures of either the tibia (shin bone) or of the bones in the feet.[2]

Running long distances is one of the biggest reasons people get injured. In men the risk of injury goes up considerably if they run more than sixty-five kilometres (forty miles) per week. This has been shown in military recruits, who are sometimes required to dramatically increase the intensity of their physical fitness regimens. Having a high foot arch (*pes cavus*) is also a big risk factor for injury, whereas most other variations in foot shape don't increase injury risk.[3]

I first learned to examine joints during our clinical exam course in my first year of medical school. During the initial few weeks, we learned how to take a patient history. We practised history-taking with "standardized patients" — actors who were paid to play out a certain scenario or diagnosis. We soon moved on to seeing real patients. Then we learned how to conduct a musculoskeletal exam — how to inspect the joint looking for swelling, redness, deformity; how to palpate to elicit tender spots; how to stress the joints to assess for ligament injuries; and how to do specialized tests to check for such things as injures to the meniscus (the soft cushion between the bones of the knee), or a rupture of the Achilles tendon.

These physical exam skills were pushed to new limits during my orthopaedic surgery rotation. We would have patients walk up and down the hall and assess their gait and the angulation of their knees. We would attend fracture clinic where orthopaedic staff and residents would move quickly from case to case, reviewing X-rays, examining the injuries, and prescribing continued splinting, casting, or — what every patient hoped for — cast removal and permission to get on with their lives. We would see patients in the emergency room with new injuries. One man broke his femur and multiple vertebrae when he lost control of his toboggan while sledding; another was hit by a taxi while cycling home from work.

Much of the time during orthopaedic or emergency medicine rotations, I would be yanking or pulling on dislocated joints to get them back in place while patients were given powerful sedatives and opioids to ensure they had minimal pain, or no memory at all of the experience. During surgery I would hold back skin flaps while the surgeon removed a diseased knee joint and replaced it with a metal and plastic prosthesis. During the procedure, the surgeon would drill me and my classmates on knee anatomy and run through clinical scenarios with us — often involving tobogganing accidents.

I reflected on my time working with orthopaedic surgeons when I read about the writer Bernd Heinrich's knee injury, which developed while he was training for the Boston Marathon:

> Soon after I started training, I got a knee pain. I went to an orthopaedic surgeon, who said, "You have some sort of cartilage degeneration. If you don't stop running, I'm going to have to

> take your kneecap off and throw it in the garbage can." His exact words. They rang in my ears a long time. I figured, instead, that I had a loose piece of cartilage, which I could get rid of by grinding it down by running, so I increased my mileage.

Bernd went on to run the Boston Marathon in 2 hours and 25 minutes and continued to run for the rest of his life including, most memorably, winning the U.S. 100K championship in Chicago in 1981.

In any given year around thirty thousand runners register for the Boston Marathon; slightly fewer than 90 percent make it to the finish line. What happens to the missing 10 percent, you may wonder? Most of those who don't cross the finish line don't even make it to the start line. My colleague Janet was one who made it to the Boston Marathon but couldn't finish. She had injured her Achilles tendon during training and hoped that her pain would settle down for the race. Within ten minutes of starting, she knew it wasn't going to be easy, and by the 13K point, she couldn't tolerate the pain and decided to drop out of the marathon and race another day.

Janet's Achilles injury, like many running injuries, began after she abruptly increased her volume of training. This is one of the biggest risk factors for any type of sports injury. The key to minimizing this risk is to increase training volumes gradually.

When Paul came to see me for his regular follow-up, I noticed he was limping. "It's my heel," he said, as I looked at him with concern.

"What happened?" I asked.

He said he didn't know, but for about three weeks, he'd had worsening pain at the back of his foot. "It's so bad I was crying."

I had known Paul for several years and would often see him walking his dog, Churchill, during my lunchtime runs on the river paths near the clinic.

"I've still been walking. I can't give that up, and Churchill needs to get out."

I knew Paul was tough. He was a veteran of life on the street who always had a new plan to make some extra cash. I couldn't imagine him crying. I looked at the bony prominence on the back of his foot, known as the posterior calcaneus. Then I felt along his Achilles tendon about three centimetres up.

"That's where it hurts," he muttered, flinching from the pain.

I asked him if the pain was burning, a common description for Achilles pain, and he nodded agreement.

"It gets worse the more I walk, but I just can't stay home. I'll go insane," he told me.

I knew his pain was occurring because of small persistent damage to the tendon. It was not healing because of recurrent use and repetitive strain.

About 10 percent of running injuries involve the Achilles tendon. Treatment is usually rest. Take a break from running, put ice on the tendon, take anti-inflammatories, and support the tendon with a heel lift or athletic tape.

One treatment that patients regularly request is the beloved cortisone injection. Many have had one before and found it led to many months of pain relief. Others have found no benefit at all. A major review that looked at thousands of patients who had steroid injections for conditions such as tennis elbow and Achilles tendinopathy found most people felt a lot better after the injection. However, after six to twelve months there were much lower rates of full recovery from the injury in those who got the injection, and their risk of returning pain and dysfunction was 63 percent higher than those who avoided the shot in favour of rest and physiotherapy.[4] Multiple other reviews have had similar findings, showing short-term benefit but long-term risks. Steroids inhibit collagen synthesis, and this may impair healing and increase the risk of tendon rupture.[5]

Janet missed out on the Boston Marathon but was back to training for an Ironman before long. Her injury was very mild compared to the ones suffered by those who push so hard that they rupture their tendon. When the Achilles tendon ruptures, the calf muscles contract up into the leg and you lose one of the most important stabilizers in your leg. This is a devastating injury that I've seen a number of times in my patients. Sprinters have the highest lifetime risk of Achilles tendon rupture.[6]

Soccer and basketball players are also at increased risk due to the extreme stresses placed on the tendon during sudden starts and stops.

Another patient, Jacob, told me about his injury. He was jumping to make a block in a pickup game of basketball when he heard a pop and felt suddenly like someone had kicked him in the back of the ankle. He looked around but there was no one there. When he tried to get up, he saw a bulge just under his knee where there hadn't been one before. He knew something bad had happened, but it was only in the emergency room an hour later that he learned what had happened — his Achilles tendon had ruptured. I saw him two weeks after his surgical repair, and he was still wearing an Aircast and walking on crutches. Although Jacob had a long rehabilitation process, soon enough he was back to regular exercise. "I just can't sit still," he told me apologetically.

Every week a patient comes in with foot pain as their chief complaint. I ask about any recent injuries, I ask about what kind of activity they do, and I look at their foot. The first diagnosis I usually consider when they say the pain is at the back of the foot is plantar fasciitis. I always ask the same question: "Does it hurt most when you get out of bed in the morning?" If they say yes and go on to say that once they get moving the pain subsides, then I start thinking about the tests I'll do to stress their feet to confirm the diagnosis. If they say no, then I take a step back and consider a wider range of options.

Runners are at risk of plantar fasciitis; it is the most common reason for a runner to develop rear foot pain. The pain is usually worse when pushing off during running or walking. We don't know for sure why it develops, but it seems to be linked to too much side-to-side movement of the foot and is more common in older and heavier runners.[7] The test that I do to confirm my suspicion is to grasp the patient's foot and bend their toes back while pressing my thumb into the soft middle of the foot. I try to be as gentle as possible then increase pressure until my patient looks like they are genuinely suffering. Of course, sometimes that isn't the problem, and they tell me that movement doesn't hurt. Then they show me that the pain is actually somewhere else in the foot.

When I make the diagnosis, I prescribe a series of stretches and exercises of the foot and toes. I tell them to stand on a big book and curl their toes over the edge then practise picking up a towel by curling their toes. They usually come back within a few weeks telling me things are better. I encourage them to see a physiotherapist for more guidance if they are still suffering.

Recently, Natalie came into my clinic complaining of pain just to the outside her right shin. "I've already diagnosed myself with a stress fracture," she said sheepishly. She then apologized for reading about her injury online.

I told her it was great: the more patients know, the better for everyone. It's much easier for me to make a diagnosis when a patient has already put thought into their symptoms and what may or may not be the cause.

I told her a stress fracture wasn't a certainty as shin pain can also be from shin splints. We decided to do an X-ray, and I suggested that she hold back on running for a few weeks to help reduce the pain. Stress fractures can be hard to diagnose; thus, even if her X-ray was negative, we might need to do other imaging like a bone scan or MRI to be certain about the diagnosis.

While Natalie had shin pain, runners are most likely to injure their knees, and the most common problem with the knee is patellofemoral syndrome, something I had experienced while ramping up my kilometres two years before. I started having a vague pain on the inside of my right knee, so I went to see Lynne, the physiotherapist at my clinic. I told her about the time I had smashed my knee playing squash, and she said I had patellofemoral syndrome probably started by that trauma. She showed me how the muscles on the inside of my knee were much weaker than on the outside.

"That imbalance in muscles and the tightness of your iliotibial band pulls the knee cap out and causes your pain," she explained.

So she sent me to the gym to learn some exercises, and within a week my pain was gone. It was my first and, so far, only personal experience with physiotherapy. I had always been a believer, but now my faith took on an even greater intensity. "Go to physio," I would advise my patients with musculoskeletal injuries, "and you will be healed." And almost always, they were.

After my own experience with patellofemoral syndrome, I started to notice more cases among my patients. They would usually complain of pain at the front their knees, which became worse after sitting for a long time, such as an extended car journey, or when going up or down stairs. Some would describe lots of strange sounds coming from their knees, like popping or clicking.[8] When I tried to understand what had led them to develop patellofemoral syndrome, they often told me similar stories of recently increasing their physical activity. In runners this almost always came from training for a race.

While most of these patients need to reduce their running volume, this is especially the case if they are really suffering. Runners with milder symptoms may get better just by cutting out some of the extreme aspects of their regime, such as hill running. They can focus on cross-training on a bicycle, swimming, or water running.[9] Focused exercises that work the medial quadriceps and stretch the iliotibial band can also be particularly helpful, as they were in my case.

While patellofemoral syndrome is the most common cause of knee pain in a runner, iliotibial band syndrome is a close second. Early in my training as a resident, a young woman named Irene came to my clinic complaining of aching pain that radiated on the outside of her knee up toward her thigh. This pain was worse when running and had been occurring more frequently in the past three months. She had never injured her knee or leg before and was frustrated that the pain was interfering with her training for an upcoming 10K run. I used some of the tests that I had learned in my physical exam course to determine if the problem was with the iliotibial band. I had her lie on her side and stress the IT band by doing a kind of scissor motion with her legs.

"That definitely hurts more," she grimaced.

I showed her a picture of the IT band and explained that it was a thick band of connective tissue running from the bony edge of the pelvic girdle called the *ilium* all the way down to the tibia just on the outside of the knee. As I described it to her, I remembered the day in first year medical school when I dissected the leg and felt the thick powerful connection formed by this shining piece of connective tissue. I told her that the IT band stabilizes the knee during running and also helps move the knee and hip.

"What can I do? Do I have to stop running?" she asked anxiously.

It is ironic that while I spend much of my time encouraging patients to run more, an unlucky few need to do the opposite and actually find it hard to be less active. With IT band syndrome, it's okay to be moderately active so long as you don't have symptoms — if you do, then you need to pull back a bit. After reducing the offending activity, the other key steps are frequent icing and using anti-inflammatories to help with the pain. Then specific exercises are used to strengthen the leg and the IT band is regularly stretched to improve mobility.

While training for a race in Amsterdam one year, I started to feel sharp pain on the outside of my right knee. It felt like someone had hit me with a lead pipe. I sat down on a bench, thought for a moment, and diagnosed myself with IT band syndrome. I put my right leg behind my left leg and bent down to touch my toes. The pain shot back, radiating up and down from my knee. *Yes,* I thought, *it's my IT band, but what does this mean for my training?* For the next few days, I stretched my IT band, rolled it on my beloved foam roller, and began the same hip-stabilizing exercises I had discussed with my patient several years before.

The next Sunday marked three weeks before the race, and with some reservation, I embarked on a long training run. Just before halfway, the pain came back. I was far from home, and I needed to get back to take my kids to their swimming lessons. I stopped running and walked through the cool morning for a few minutes. A place that was normally the most gloriously uplifting stretch of nature on the Ottawa River seemed remote and hostile. My mind was churning through my options, including that of abandoning my run and summoning an Uber to get home. After a few minutes of walking, the pain subsided, and I decided to try a little gentle running.

For the next hour I ran home in a moderate amount of pain. I knew my few days of stretching and exercise hadn't been enough to fix a problem that had likely been developing over the past several months. During that time I had dramatically increased my training distance. So for the next two weeks I kept my distance down, and every day, instead of going on a long run, I gingerly jogged ten minutes to my local park, where I faithfully performed my self-prescribed stretches and exercises. The week before the race, I ran fast for eleven kilometres. It was to be the test as to whether I was fit to compete. At the end of the run I felt gloriously happy; I was euphoric, after having gone so long without my customary runner's high. But the test, like so many in medicine, was not definitive. I had felt in great shape, but toward the end of the run, I did feel a twinge in my IT band.

The next morning I woke up remembering a dream I had in which I was scheduled to run the Olympic marathon but couldn't find my shoes, socks, or the way to the start line. It was a classic anxiety dream — like when someone dreams they have a big exam the next day but have completely forgotten to study. I rested a few days then decided I was ready. I travelled to Amsterdam and pinned my race number to my shirt.

Race day was October 15. I gave myself two and a half hours to travel from my mother's house in the medieval town of Delft to the start line in Amsterdam. My planned train was cancelled, but I adjusted my route, and as I sprinted out of the station to catch the last bus, I felt a sense of calm at having made it just under the wire. My relief was clouded over, however, as the minutes elapsed with no sight of the Olympic stadium where the race was to begin. I spotted a small crowd of passengers in athletic wear urgently negotiating with the bus driver. A red-haired woman looked at the racing number pinned to my chest and explained in an Irish accent that the marathon had resulted in this bus taking a detour that would leave us nowhere near the start line. A young blond woman who was anxiously gripping a stroller in one hand and looking intently at her phone exclaimed, "We're thirteen kilometres from the stadium."

The race was to start in twenty-five minutes. A tall young man wearing black running tights said that the driver had agreed to drop us off on the exit from the highway.

We emerged from the bus onto an industrial street in the outskirts of Amsterdam. I had no functioning phone, so I was at the mercy of my fellow racers, who began to walk hastily down the sidewalk. A minute later we were running. With a detached sense of amusement, I wondered if the plan was to run the thirteen kilometres to the start line. The Irishwoman and her husband jogged slowly behind us while the woman with her stroller urgently pushed it forward. After a few hundred metres we arrived at a Metro station. I realized that we had been running because our train was about to arrive. We boarded just in time, and in only ten minutes, we stepped out at the Olympic stadium. After weeks of ambivalence about this race, I felt elated to have arrived, to not have this race stolen from me by the vagaries of chance and the Amsterdam public transport system. I waved goodbye to my fellow passengers, all of whom still had to pick up their race kits before they could join me at the start line.

I walked slowly toward my holding area as the marathoners streamed into the Olympic stadium to our side. It was a sunny day, but it was fresh and not nearly as humid as Ottawa had been for the past several months. We started moving slowly toward the start line as people cheered and watched from their balconies and behind the barricades erected on the street. After ten minutes we started running. Although I had been to Amsterdam as a child, my only memory of that trip was seeing a Nintendo console and playing *Super Mario Bros.* for the very first time. Now twenty-five years later and surrounded by tens of thousands of runners, I began my 21.1-kilometre tour. We moved quickly along tree-lined avenues and streamed onto bridges over canals. We passed cyclists in the thousands. At points, the path narrowed to only a few metres forcing us to squeeze together and slow slightly as the juggernaut of runners edged forward.

At the first water station I reached for a white bar from a volunteer's outstretched hand and bit into the morsel cautiously. It was some kind of bland nougat with almonds. I decided it must be a Dutch superfood and ate the rest quickly. At the next few stations I tried lemon and then orange Isostar electrolyte drink, remembering both times why I had chosen water as my training drink. At the final stations I reached for big pieces of bananas instead of nougat. We passed the grand Rijksmuseum and the Heineken brewery, and then turned into a beautiful park filled with cheering spectators.

I felt light on my feet, having not run at all in five days and only very little in the weeks before that. So at sixteen kilometres I thought of Roger Bannister's strong kick in the final moments of a race and decided to push hard on the accelerator. This was a mistake. After a few glorious seconds of my kick, I felt the lead pipe strike my right knee. I grimaced and slowed down, then I slowed down some more, and then I was limping slightly, waiting for the pain to pass.

I needed to stay mentally strong. I imagined going for my favourite 5K run around Dow's Lake. I imagined that at the end of the run I'd come home to my family. I imagined hearing my daughter yell "Papa" and run to the door to show me the picture she was drawing. I imagined my son building Lego and my wife sitting peacefully drinking her coffee. I was inspired by Paula Radcliffe, one of history's best marathoners, who would say her children's names to herself to keep up her unbreakable spirit in the painful moments of a race.

In a few moments my pain stopped, and I was able to get back to a comfortable pace. We passed a long road flanked by cafes, turned right, and were suddenly back at the Olympic stadium. After reading about the history of the Olympics, this moment was one of the reasons I had chosen to come to this city and run this race. The Amsterdam Olympics of 1928 was one of the great early demonstrations of the special allure of this international festival of sport, and I was racing on hallowed ground.

We entered the stadium filled with spectators and pushed around the track toward the finish line. I felt I had not given everything to the race as I protected my injury, but I was so happy to be done. I jogged slowly to catch the train back to Delft. On the train I was somnolent, drifting off to sleep until the conductor, after asking for my ticket, pointed to my race bib and said something to me in Dutch. When I made it clear I didn't understand, he asked in English, "How was your race?" I told him I'd had fun and he nodded knowingly before saying, "That's important" in his clipped Dutch accent.

I was scheduled to run another half-marathon three weeks later, but I knew that I needed to let my IT band heal. I planned to start icing it at night and redouble my strengthening exercises. I wanted to keep running so badly. I could relate even more to my patients through the years who were so afraid of being told that the best treatment for their running injury was to stop running.

Of course, some people don't have a choice. Carla told me about the terrible knee pain that had started after she abruptly changed direction during a soccer practice.

"I heard a pop and my whole knee felt bad right away," she told me.

She drove to the emergency room and limped up to the triage nurse. After a few hours she had an MRI which showed a complete rupture of her anterior cruciate ligament (ACL). She was seen by the orthopedic surgery team and before long she had a surgical repair of her ACL. It was a frightening experience for her, her first time in an operating room, her first time sleeping in a hospital. I saw her recently in follow-up, and she told me it had been the most painful year of her life. First the injury, then the post-op pain, then months of rehab and home exercises. She had also gained weight, which she was working hard to lose by changing her diet and increasing her exercise.

As I was running later that day, I thought about how much pain that one "pop" had caused Carla. It's frustrating to see people who are trying to stay fit and active get injured doing the thing they love, even if that's parkour. It was a beautiful January morning and the Rideau Canal was open for skating, so I decided to do my long run on the snowy edge. For the first few kilometres I was very cautious, but I soon found that the surface was hardly slippery at all. It felt amazing to run on the fine snowy top layer, which was soft and forgiving and looked like sand in the bright winter sun.

Every winter the staff in the emergency department of the nearby Civic Hospital brace themselves for an onslaught of victims of the frozen canal. Usually, people who haven't been skating in a while or get a bit too exuberant end up falling on outstretched hands and breaking a wrist or landing hard and snapping an ankle bone. At night, the light is minimal, so the cracks or small potholes that form during the day are difficult to discern, and the unsuspecting skater can fall pretty hard. I've suffered a few big falls, but so far I haven't ended up in the emergency room.

Every time a runner laces up and puts on winter gloves and a hat, they are risking a bad slip on the ice. A colleague in my clinic told me a cautionary tale of her friend who fell while running in the winter: the woman fractured her tibia and fibula and was unable to run for six months afterward. These are sobering stories, and they do give me pause. I pause for a moment until I realize the alternative to running in winter conditions is not running. The question is how to prevent injury whether running on ice, on a trail, or on dry tarmac.

Let's start with a simple way people often try to prevent injury: warming up. Warming up sounds like a good idea; many of my training runs begin with five or ten minutes of slow jogging. However, studies that have looked at teaching runners a standardized program for warming up and cooling down have not been able to show any reduction in the injury rate. This hasn't prevented me from starting most runs at a gentle pace, mostly because it feels right, and it lets me mentally and physically prepare for the tougher parts of a training run.

Now, consider stretching. Again, studies have not really been able to show that stretching before or after a workout reduces injuries. However, what studies have shown is that people who stretch feel better. A study of nine hundred military recruits suggested that those who stretched regularly experienced lower rates of low back and other soft tissue pain.[10] Of course, I do believe specific stretches treat certain conditions like plantar fasciitis, Achilles tendonitis, and IT band syndrome, but so far, the evidence doesn't suggest the practice can prevent injuries.

What about shoes? One thing we know for sure is that older shoes provide less protection against the pounding forces experienced during running. New shoes lose up to half their shock absorption properties after 250 to 500 running miles. So changing your shoes at least every five hundred miles makes sense. A study of participants in the Vancouver Sun Run 10K race showed that men whose shoes were more than four months old had higher rates of injury. For women, the increased risk occurred once their shoes were more than six months old. The theory here is that men are heavier and thus wear out their shoes faster.[11] Along with new shoes, insoles and orthotics can also help. Another trial among military trainees found that those given customized orthotics had significantly fewer overuse injuries in their legs and feet. Orthotics probably also reduce the risk of stress fractures in the foot, and they reduce the pain associated with patellofemoral syndrome and high arched feet.[12]

What about barefoot running? It's hard to open a running magazine without seeing an article or advertisement promoting barefoot or minimalist running. While my brother Sascha embraced the movement years ago and had an excellent experience, I have yet to make the switch. The most widely cited paper on barefoot running was published by Daniel Lieberman and his colleagues in the journal *Nature* in 2010. On Lieberman's website there is a photo of him with his intellectual beard, wearing a red tech shirt and grey shorts, and running barefoot across one of the bridges crossing the Charles River in Boston. In the photo, the great man is smiling while his left foot hovers a few centimetres above the ground.

The *Nature* article is impressive to read. It begins with the observation that "[h]umans have engaged in endurance running for millions of years, but the modern running shoe was not invented until the 1970s. For most of human evolutionary history, runners were either barefoot or wore minimal footwear such as sandals or moccasins with smaller heels and little cushioning relative to modern running shoes."[13]

The key difference between a barefoot and shod runner is how they land during foot strike — shod runners tend to land on their heels while barefoot runners tend to land on their forefeet. The mantra among barefoot activists is that the forefoot strike is good and heel strike is bad.

Up to 80 percent of shod runners land on the rear of their feet, a habit made possible and perhaps inevitable by the design of modern running shoes. Most shoes have a large heel built of materials designed to absorb and redistribute the impact of rear foot strike. On the other hand, runners who are brought up training barefoot or who make the switch to barefoot often land on their forefeet. The key to the argument that this is a "superior" form of running is that forefoot strikers "generate smaller collision force than shod rear-foot strikers."[14]

As expected from Lieberman, the group makes an evolutionary argument, contending that "if endurance running was an important behaviour before the invention of modern shoes," we would have evolved the anatomy and running style that minimized injury when barefoot or in minimal footwear.[15] They also speculate that barefoot running may lead to less injury because of reduced impact during each of the six hundred foot strikes per kilometre. They criticize cushioned running shoes for limiting proprioception and encouraging the much maligned rear foot strike.

When Adharanand Finn was planning his trip to Kenya, he decided to adopt a barefoot style. He threw out his running shoes and spoke to leaders in the field, changed his running form, and slowly rebuilt himself as a runner. Should the rest of us do the same?

There are many differences between barefoot and shod runners beyond just what is covering their feet. There are differences in gait, stride length, and, as discussed, which part of the foot strikes the ground first. Based on Lieberman's arguments, it is logical to assume that stress on the joints would be less with proper barefoot form, and therefore injury rates would be lower. One study found that barefoot running reduced the peak stresses experienced by the patellofemoral joint by 12 percent compared to shod running.[16]

A study published in the *British Journal of Sports Medicine* in 2015 examined injury rates between barefoot and shod runners. Over the course of a year, the investigators followed 201 adult runners — roughly half of whom were barefoot runners and half of whom were shod runners. Every month the runners logged their miles and any injuries. The study found that the injury rate per mile run was the same between the two groups, although the types of injuries differed. Barefoot runners hurt the soles of their feet more and had more calf injuries, while shod runners had more knee injuries and more plantar fasciitis.[17] Other studies have also suggested more stress fractures of the foot in those running with minimalist footwear.[18]

Another important study, published in 2017, found that heavy runners suffered more with barefoot running than lighter runners, and that more running led to more injuries.[19] Sixty-one runners were randomly assigned to two different shoe types: minimalist or regular running shoes. Over twenty-six weeks, the runners all gradually increased their training distances. Runners in minimalist shoes were more likely to be injured, and minimalist runners weighing more than eighty-five kilograms were much more likely to be injured. Some clinicians therefore recommend that heavier runners stick with conventional running shoes.[20] Thus, while barefoot running is for many a delightful way to change and refresh their running experience, it is not a panacea.

Sometimes sports medicine is less science than art, thus runners get conflicting advice from different sources. I believe that there is no one correct way to run. I remember this point being driven home while watching two women race to the finish line of a recent London Marathon. One woman was nearly six feet tall and had a long loping gait; the other was small and ran with shorter, more rapid steps. Their bodies were moving so differently that the only thing you could confidently say was that they were both running. And yet they were two of the fastest runners in the world, reaching the top of a gruelling competition with very different biological endowments and very different styles. Trying to change your running form can be challenging. I have seen evidence that the longer you run, the more efficient your style becomes; forcing yourself into a different form can actually reduce your efficiency.[21] Finding your own way is a better approach than being prescribed a specific type of running form.

I was taken aback by a running statistic recently — there are twenty-four thousand emergency room visits in the United States every year resulting from accidents on treadmills.[22] Having been catapulted off a treadmill a few times, I can appreciate the inherent danger of these machines.

A fellow runner asked me a few years ago if I like running on treadmills. I was emphatic in my lack of enthusiasm. "It's nothing like the running I know," I emphasized.

She agreed, telling me, "The boredom is indescribable."

For many runners, the only reason to run on a treadmill is because you can't run outside, and if you learn to love running in all weather, there is never a day when you can't run outside. Unless you live in New

Delhi. I learned that during an addiction medicine conference in India when the pollution and traffic kept me from going outside and I had to stick with the treadmill.

But one innovation I have used more recently has made treadmill running really fun. Instead of watching the dreary news, the treadmill's screen gave me the option to run a simulated trail from a choice of beautiful trails from around the world. I chose to run through the German forest while my son tried a New Zealand coastal trail. It wasn't quite virtual reality, just a video of the trail moving in front of me, but the mind can be easily tricked, and as I ran on the treadmill, I imagined myself on the forest trail. I really did feel good after running. Placebo? Perhaps, but it worked.

Running on treadmills is very gentle on the joints, and running surface does seem to alter a runner's risk of injury. One of the big differences Adharanand Finn noted on his travels to Kenya and then Japan was the difference in surfaces preferred. The Kenyans ran almost exclusively on dirt trails while the Japanese ran predominantly on paved roads. The Stanford biomechanics researcher Katherine Boyer suggests that flat, uniform surfaces increase the risk of injury because each stride will be almost identical, thus resulting in repetitive strain–type injuries on muscles, bones, and joints.[23] The Kenyan experience of slightly uneven terrain may reduce the risk of injury because each step is slightly different, thus spreading out the stress more diffusely through the impacted areas. Most runners I know prefer to avoid paved roads as much as possible, but trail running comes with the risks of falling and spraining an ankle. I had several close calls during my first trail race in Gatineau Park, and I witnessed a nasty fall on a downhill stretch.

Other types of injuries can befall athletes, harms that don't leave a bruise or a scar. I was reminded of this one spring morning when I saw a thirty-five-year-old man in my clinic who complained of fatigue. But he was not like other patients with that common complaint. Most people are tired, overweight, and sedentary. Maybe they have sleep apnea, diabetes, or are just out of shape. But this man, Calvin, was different. He was tall and strong. He told me he began to feel tired a few months into training for an ultramarathon that was coming up in Montana. He was a serious runner, and when I probed a little further into how hard he was training, he admitted that he wasn't training to compete; he was training to win, as he had done at numerous ultra races in recent years.

We reviewed his recent blood tests including hemoglobin, vitamin B12, iron, thyroid, and blood sugar — they were all normal. We explored his symptoms a bit more — he was tired but couldn't get to sleep at night. His heart rate was shooting up from his normally low resting heart rate of fifty-five beats per minute. And when he did try to train, he felt like his limbs were huge and heavy. He'd even suffered a respiratory infection a few weeks earlier that took longer than usual to clear.

When I raised the possible diagnosis of overtraining syndrome, Calvin told me he'd been thinking along similar lines but had never experienced these symptoms in the past. His whole athletic life, he had pushed his body harder and harder to reach high levels of athletic ability.

Training is all about putting greater stresses on the body as it adapts to prior training loads in order to force the body to higher levels of performance.[24] You overload your body, then expect to have a period of fatigue during which the body regenerates with rest and the right blend of carbohydrates and protein. Then you hit your body again and again, repeatedly overloading it and willing your muscles to compensate and super-compensate as they strengthen and as your endurance grows.

But in order to recover, the body needs at least four key factors: hydration, nutrition, physical rest, and sleep.[25] When any one or more of the key recovery factors is missing, athletes can develop overtraining syndrome. Overtraining syndrome is characterized by a decline in performance associated with fatigue, moodiness, infections, and a feeling of burnout lasting for two or more months. And overtraining is common. I have seen a number of new runners who are so excited to have found running that they just keep going and run themselves straight into overtraining syndrome. Around six out of every ten runners will experience overtraining syndrome in their lifetime.

When I talked about managing his symptoms, Calvin and I skirted around the most obvious treatment, which was to stop training. No athlete wants to hear those words, and running lore is filled with tales of runners who were told they should or would never run again but who go on to overcome their injuries to achieve new heights of glory. Instead, we talked about less drastic options, such as reducing the intensity of his training for two weeks and then reassessing. Calvin struggled with lower levels of activity but quickly noticed his mood improving and his energy coming back.

If too much exercise can make you feel tired, can it also make you sick? Moderately active individuals typically have a lower risk of upper respiratory infections compared with sedentary individuals, but beyond a certain point, as activity level continues to increase, so does risk. One possible explanation for this is the "open window theory," which posits that the immune system is temporarily impaired for a few hours after an intense workout leading to a "window" of opportunity for viruses to infect the athlete.[26]

The medications that athletes use to combat such infections can be harmful. Older antihistamines like Benadryl can increase the risk of heat illness and dehydration and can also cause sedation. Second-generation antihistamine formulations are less sedating but can still be dehydrating. Cough suppressants like dextromethorphan can make you feel tired, while decongestants can also increase the risks of dehydration and overheating.[27]

So, putting all this together, how can runners avoid injuries? First, runners will have fewer injuries if they keep their total training distance to less than sixty-five kilometres per week. They should also stagger intense stresses on their bodies. For example, long runs (more than twenty kilometres) should be done no more than every two weeks. It's probably best not to run every day. Runners should probably take one rest day and one or two cross-training days. Finally, there is the issue of how much to race. A marathon puts a lot of stress on the body, and it's probably in your best interest to avoid running more than two or three marathons per year, but these limits will differ based on a person's age, injury history, and genetics.[28]

Slowly building up intensity can help reduce a variety of injuries, including overtraining syndrome. Wearing comfortable shoes well-suited to your foot structure or wearing minimalist shoes with close supervision will help. Running on a soft surface and avoiding fast downhill runs will reduce strain on your joints. Strengthening programs focused on quadriceps and hip muscles also reduce the risk of injury. Furthermore, calf exercises designed to protect the Achilles tendon may reduce the risk of tendon injury, particularly as you get older.[29]

Finally, nutrition and hydration are important. My father learned this the hard way after standing up from bed, fainting, and hitting his head on a table as he came down. After he saw a cardiologist and took some tests, his doctor suggested he needed to take in more electrolytes and fluid after exercising. Eating carbohydrates and protein within thirty minutes of an intense workout also helps with tissue repair.[30]

So many factors need to come together to keep your body healthy enough to start running, to train to improve, to achieve your peak fitness, to race your best times, or just to keep lacing up week after week as you work to keep your body fit and strong despite the vagaries of aging.

When I suffer from running on city streets, I find myself hearing the wild call of the trail run ever louder. One afternoon I was sitting in my addiction medicine clinic and four patients failed to show up for their appointments. This is not so unusual, as missing appointments is a symptom of a bad addiction. So I used the time to read about a race of which I had only heard whispers, La Chute du Diable. It is a trail race held in a national park outside of Montreal. My heart quickened and my pupils dilated as I looked at the map of the race. Eighty kilometres on trails with 2,800 metres of elevation. Impossible. Then I saw there is also a 50K race with 1,500 metres of elevation. Could it be done?

Of course, the human body is a miracle. I know that. Every year runners compete in, and finish, the Marathon des Sables, a six-day, 251-kilometre race through the Sahara Desert. They run in desert heat; they run a marathon every day for six days in a row. In 1994 a sandstorm wreaked havoc on the race. An Italian Olympian named Mauro Prosperi ended up almost three hundred kilometres off course and was lost for eleven days in the desert. And yet every year more endurance warriors return to race in the desert.

As I thought of La Chute du Diable, my brain went into overdrive: How would I train? How would I protect my iliotibial band? What would happen on race day? What could I carry with me? How amazing would it feel to run alone on those beautiful mountain trails for eighty kilometres? How would it change me, change my brain? There came a knock at the door. A patient had arrived. I pushed all thought of trail ultramarathons out of my mind. First, I needed to ready myself for the entry exam to the club of runners; first, I needed to run a marathon.

VIII RUNNING A MARATHON

I decided to fly to Berlin for my first marathon. Of all the major marathons in the world, Berlin called loudest. I watched the previous races online. The race starts in the Tiergarten, steps from the German parliament's new home in the Reichstag and ends at the Brandenburg Gate. I read online how much other runners love this race and often come back many times.

Why run a marathon? For most contemporary runners, the marathon stands as a monolith towering above other events in the running landscape. Historically, it was the heavy weight, the beast that knew no peer. Its call brings millions to run in marathons every year around the world. We are taught to believe that to be a real runner, you must run at least one marathon.

There will always be contenders to the throne. A few years ago, I saw a running magazine with the headline "Is 100 miles the new marathon?"

I found this question delightful. It spoke to me about the boundless ambition of runners and of our species. If we can do better or go farther, we will. The article made me think of the debate about whether humans should colonize Mars. One argument traces humanity back to Africa and our movement from there to all corners of the globe, noting our urge to travel and expand our horizons, to explore undiscovered country.

Dopamine may also be implicated. Although the genetic research has not been conclusive, dopamine and dopamine receptors seem to be involved in novelty-seeking. It may be the case that people with certain types of genes or personality traits are more likely to leave the safety and comfort of home to journey to unknown lands. Similarly, people who choose to run ultramarathons or travel to Mars likely have some combination of genes that push them to explore beyond ordinary experience.

I realized Pete Kostelnick likely has some beneficial genetic mutation after reading about his world record run across the United States, from San Francisco City Hall to New York City Hall.[1] He completed the run in October 2016 after 42 days, 6 hours, and 30 minutes of running, beating the previous record set in 1980 by four days. A run such as this, like many extreme sports, inspires us to push ourselves beyond our comfortable limits, to seek out new challenges and new adventures. But for now, the marathon is a sufficient challenge for most of us. And while running marathons may be prosaic in the running community, only a small percentage of people will ever accomplish or wish to accomplish such a feat.

The stories of ancient Greece are interwoven with stories of runners. In *The Odyssey*, Homer describes Achilles as the "fleet-footed hero" competing at funeral games. The first Olympic Games were held as a competition between the Greek city states around 700 BCE. The Games began with a sprint over the length of the stadium with the runners carrying torches to light the flame on the altar of Zeus.[2] The Olympic Games and the ancient Greek view of sport and game celebrated physical fitness and the human body.

The Olympic Games faded away with the decline of Classical Greece and only recurred as a concept in the 1890s. The Olympics were reborn with the moto *Citius, Altius, Fortius* — faster, higher, stronger. Early in its modern history, a race was created to commemorate the messenger's run from Marathon to Athens with news of the victory over the Persians in 490 BCE.[3] The very first marathon retracing this journey was held in 1895. It began on the Plain of Marathon and ended at the newly built Olympic Stadium in Athens, a distance of twenty-five miles, just short of the modern marathon distance of 26.2 miles. That first race was won by Spyridon Louis, a Greek stable boy who completed the race in 2 hours, 58 minutes, 50 seconds, collapsing soon after he crossed the finish line.[4]

The next marathon was held in Paris in 1896. From there the event spread in popularity across Europe and the United States. The first Boston Marathon was held in 1897 and was designed to commemorate the ride of Paul Revere and William Dawes, who warned of the approaching British troops during the Revolutionary War.[5] The Boston Marathon was wildly popular and by 1902 was attracting crowds of at least one hundred thousand, making it the world's most watched sporting event at the time.[6]

At the London Olympic Games of 1908, the current marathon distance of 26.2 miles was established. Apparently, this occurred because the Princess of Wales wanted her children to watch the start of the race; thus, the start line was moved inside the grounds of Windsor Castle.[7]

The first London Olympic Marathon also saw the first concerns about the possible harm those who run in long races could suffer. These were spurred by the dramatic collapse of the lead runner, an Italian named Dorando Pietri, just yards from the finish line. He fell then pulled himself back up when he saw the next runner enter the stadium, only to collapse again just three yards from the finish line. In the end he was helped across the finish line. After some discussion, the second runner, an American called John Hayes, was declared the winner as he did not receive any assistance.

Today, with one-hundred-mile races becoming more commonplace, very few serious runners consider the marathon a dangerous distance, but we do see the toll it takes on our bodies and the need for specialized knowledge around fluid, electrolyte, and carbohydrate consumption during a marathon, as during any strenuous physical activity.

The first New York City Marathon was held on September 13, 1970. One hundred and twenty-six runners started the race, but only fifty completed it. Runners sweated it out during four loops around Central Park. The first marathon in Ottawa was held in 1975 and started at Carleton University. With 159 runners, it was Canada's largest marathon at the time, and it continues to be the largest — it attracts almost fifty thousand participants across a number of events every year.

From the beginning of the year, I had seen Berlin as my goal. To build up my training, I planned to run a half-marathon in May. I looked at the options and found a half-marathon trail run just outside of Ottawa, beginning in the quaint village of Wakefield and traversing the Gatineau forest. It looked perfect. What follows are my training journals for the six-month period leading up to Berlin. I have left them in their original format to capture the immediacy of the experiences.

APRIL 23

It is Saturday morning and I've just completed my last long run before the Wakefield half-marathon two weeks from today. My training has been going very well. I just came back from a week with my family in Montreal. I discovered a fourteen-kilometre trail along the Lachine Canal from the Old Port to Lake Saint-Louis. The canal has a faded industrial feel with abandoned warehouses slowly giving way to new housing developments. It is a wonderful place to train. I have loved Montreal since moving there to complete my undergrad degree at McGill and I find myself continually drawn back to the city. I met my wife at McGill and each time we visit we can't stop talking about our dream of owning a small flat on the Lachine Canal and spending as many weekends and as much of the summer there as possible.

We had been in Montreal this time to celebrate my birthday and three days later my son's birthday. On the evening of my son's birthday we walked through the Old Port and found a table in the beautiful courtyard of Jardin Nelson and listened to live jazz. We all left feeling the magic of Montreal. Yesterday morning I ran before we packed up to leave. Everyone was still sleeping, and I slipped on my running tights and bright red top and made my way to the elevators. I was barely awake, but I knew that after a few minutes of running all the sleep would desert me.

It was cool, only a few degrees above freezing, but after months running in the snow and ice, I hardly noticed it. It was raining lightly. I listened to an audiobook on the history of the atomic bomb project and ran down the grand part of McGill College Avenue past neoclassical buildings built at the height of the British Empire and declaring their roles as Customs and Port Authority buildings, with newer signs designating them as federal government agencies. I got to the Lachine Canal and ran along the canal path, focusing on my breathing, keeping my stride length steady.

As I reached the halfway point and turned around, I felt conscious of the fact that we were going home and I would not have a chance to run in Montreal until I returned for an addiction medicine meeting in October. I thought about what I would learn and who I would meet at that event. My awareness of my surroundings was elevated. I noticed an abandoned house with a strange overhanging room extending over the canal path. The side of the house was covered in graffiti in French. I couldn't make out any meaning, but it reminded me of the graffiti I had seen on pictures of the Berlin Wall. How many weeks until Berlin? I remembered the count down on the Marathon website; it was just over twenty-two weeks.

MAY 6

Today was the Wakefield trail half-marathon. I ran with my friend Dan, who is a very strong runner. It was our first time running a race together. It was an unusually warm spring day, but much of the time we were running through forest and shaded from the morning sun.

We didn't know what to expect, which was for the best as the first kilometre was up a steep ski hill, picking our way through mud, rocky patches, and little streams. The path was narrow, and there were sharper turns and steeper hills than I had ever run before. The downhill portions were just as challenging, as we plunged down dirt or gravel trails.

It took a few kilometres to warm up and get used to the uneven terrain. By the halfway point, we were both getting into our stride. For the next eight kilometres the trail levelled out and we were able to pick up our pace. At one point, we shot out of the forest and were running on the spine of a grassy hill, gently descending back toward the base. I felt the runner's heightened sense of reality. Minutes later we were back in the forest passing a runner who didn't want to let us by, urging herself to go faster, her face grimacing with the effort. As we sped down a hill, she lost her footing and tumbled to the ground, catching herself with her hands. We stopped to check on her — two doctors in the forest with no tools. She got up, told us she was unhurt, and kept running

During the race I experimented with eating on the run. I had tried a variety of foods during my training the previous summer: Clif Bars, Vector bars, frozen fruit, chocolate-covered raisins, bananas, muesli, pitas, and pretzels. I knew that I could consume thirty to sixty grams of carbohydrates per hour of racing with little gastrointestinal distress. Last year I had eaten a full dinner of fish and chips and immediately gone on a fast 10K training run, so I knew the risk of abdominal pain was low, but this was my first time eating during a race. The day before I had watched an online video demonstrating how to safety-pin a Ziploc bag into the inside of your shorts for easy access to food during a race. I had never done this during training, so I was a little worried the plastic would rip. Dan laughed at me while he carefully chewed through six apricots in two hours and I ate an entire muesli pita and a Clif Bar. There were no adverse effects, although I was quite thirsty until I reached the next water station.

Studies have shown that there is a fascinating way to trick the brain when eating during a long race. When muscles are depleted of glycogen, putting a drink with carbohydrate in your mouth, swishing it around, then spitting it out, can actually improve performance. The theory is that the brain detects the sugar, thinks more food is on the way, and, thus, recruits more muscles or communicates with them more efficiently.[8] This doesn't work early in the race when you still have lots of glycogen reserves, but later on, when it's too late to absorb more nutrition, it can be a way to shave seconds off the final kilometres and was investigated for the sub–two-hour marathon programs.

Dan and I ran together until the last few hundred metres, when he pushed ahead at the end and finished fourteen seconds before me. I raised my head and my arms as I crossed the finish line. The online photos showed me smiling, my feet floating just above the ground.

We had not hit the wall and finished just as we expended the last of our glycogen supply. Was it the carbohydrates we had methodically chewed as we raced up and down the hilly trail? Which had been more effective — the apricots or my more generous buffet? Dan had beaten me, but I didn't feel it was the apricots that made the difference.

The winner of our race was an eighteen-year-old named Aidan, but seven of the top ten runners were in the 40–49 category. At thirty-four, I knew my best races were still ahead of me.

MAY 9

Three days after the race I went online and started a new marathon training plan. It was a twenty-week plan with five runs a week making what I took to be a symbolic one hundred runs. The longest would be over three hours. Today I did a forty-minute gentle run along the Rideau River. When I finished, I knew that I had passed another milestone — the first training run for the marathon.

MAY 11

I just finished the second run in my marathon training plan. It was a one-hour gentle run through the Arboretum and the Fletcher Wildlife Garden. Yesterday I ran along the Rideau River for forty-five minutes. I almost stopped halfway through today's run. It's only been four days since my half-marathon trail run and I felt a rest wouldn't be wrong. After two minutes of thinking like this, I decided to complete the full sixty minutes and went on to finish feeling strong. I'm sitting outside in the garden now listening to birdsong. It's May 11, and according to the Berlin Marathon website, there are nineteen weeks, three days, and sixteen hours until the race begins.

JUNE 2

Over the next week I ticked off each subsequent training run — three down, ninety-seven to go — five down, nine-five to go. Ten days after the Wakefield race, I did a one-hour training run right after lunch. I changed into running shorts as it had finally started to warm up and headed out the door. I felt stiff and sore and took a while to warm up. Forty minutes into the run, I ate my first energy gel, which had the consistency of watered-down honey and gave me a rush of speed.

It was an overcast afternoon. The landscape was finally coming to full bloom with daisies spilling out across the grass and magnolia trees in full flower. I ran along the beach at Dow's Lake and saw a group of toddlers playing in the sand with buckets and shovels. At the athletic facility there was a high school track meet and a man's voice over the loudspeaker announced the start of the relay race followed by the sound of the starting pistol. Muscular teens warmed up by throwing javelins next to the track. I passed the waterfall at Hog's Back, formed by the Rideau River shooting through a dam. I saw a group of twenty young men in military uniforms sitting in a circle on the grass. Several had removed their black boots and socks after the long march from their barracks downtown.

The run was exactly ten kilometres, and when I got home, the house was eerily quiet. I had a few free hours before picking up my kids from school and then going to a dinner talk on aging. I spent some time in my study, reading and writing, picked up the kids, made dinner, and headed out for the lecture.

JUNE 9

Almost a week later it was a holiday Monday, and we packed up the car and drove forty-five minutes north into Quebec to the beach at Lac Philippe. The lake was surrounded by forest covering small hills through which I'd run the trail race a few weeks before.

I was scheduled that day for my tenth training run, a one-hour progression workout. I had been looking forwarding to getting back on the trails all weekend. Just as my wife was about to serve lunch, I headed into the forest on a trail that traced the edge of the lake for a kilometre before turning into a narrow dirt track used by campers. I was ready for the hills, sprinting down the gradient, slicing my arms, deciding not to fear the rocky hill but to embrace it.

It was like free-falling.

The path levelled out and I kept pushing, using the momentum to keep up my speed. When I came to the next hill, I embraced the altitude, this time digging in the balls of my feet as I climbed. At one point, there were a hundred wooden stairs built into the muddy hill, which I sprinted up until I came to a sign for the Laflèche Caves.

I turned around at the top of the staircase and again, believing I would not fall, raced back down. The gravel trail felt soft and forgiving. Occasionally, I would come across a group of hikers who, on seeing me coming down the narrow trail would yell "runner" and all stand back to let me pass. I got back to the beach and deliriously ate the delicious sandwiches and fruit we had brought from the city. My son was building a sandcastle with his aunt; my daughter was resisting her nap. I was drenched in euphoria.

JUNE 15

I had a long run scheduled for today. It was the twenty-seventh run in my marathon plan, and the countdown clock said it was fourteen weeks and three days until Berlin. To mix things up, I tried something new. Instead of running in the afternoon, I ate dinner with my family, then as the kids were going to bed, I slipped out the door with my water backpack on and started running. I headed through the neighbourhood toward the Rideau River. I ran along the river path toward downtown. It was around 8:00 p.m. and the sun was still high.

I ran under the highway overpass and into the neighbourhood of Vanier. I stopped to pick up Dan at his house and we ran together for the next six kilometres. He told me about the bird nest stuck in his fume hood vent, and we talked about his work at the hospital. We made a loop through Strathcona Park, where the lights were just coming on as dusk settled. As we returned close to his house, I bid him farewell and continued back home. At that point I had gone fourteen kilometres, and the large dinner I had eaten was starting to weigh me down. I drank some water and slowed my pace.

My legs felt heavy, but I had no choice but to keep putting one foot in front of the other. It was after 9:00 p.m. and my wife texted me, "Are you ok?" I reassured her that I was homeward bound. There were still four kilometres to go. Families were out in large groups strolling along the river, many of them carrying sundaes from Dairy Queen. They looked at me with mild interest as I staggered past, dripping with sweat. I imagined them asking, *Who is this guy and what's that thing on his back?* I pushed on, crossing the bridge, and noted how low the water was for this time of year. It had rained only a few times this spring and across the city ponds and rivers were drier than in previous years.

I got back to my street and stopped running. I walked the last few minutes home, mindful of my body. The tightness in my right Achilles tendon, the dull ache in my knee, my full stomach. I went inside, drank a glass of ice water, and lay on the floor. I had no runner's high. I felt spent, wasted by the effort. Was I overtraining? I thought of my patient struggling to train, unable to find his usual strength. I had been fighting off a bad cough and sinusitis that had affected the whole family over the preceding two weeks. It had gotten much warmer as well.

The next morning I felt sore. My right Achilles tendon was so tight it felt like it was snapping around when I walked. My knee felt fine, but I knew I needed to rest. At work I talked to my student Keith about overtraining. Keith had emailed me a couple of months earlier asking to work with me before he finished residency as he wanted to have some experience in addiction medicine. The first day I met him, I was surprised by how big he was. I also noticed he was older than the other residents who usually came to my clinic. I asked him what his background was, and it all made sense. He told me he went to McGill as an undergraduate, but his real passion was judo. He went to four Olympic Games on the Canadian judo team and won a gold at the Pan American Games. After his athletic career, he had looked around at his options and decided to pursue medicine.

Whenever he was in the clinic and someone came in with a musculoskeletal injury, I got Keith to take a look. He told me that when he would train for the Olympics he would push himself as far as possible but learned to walk the fine line between burning brightly and burning out. "Guys would overtrain all the time," he said. When this happened, they would pull back and wait for their strength to return, then they would push again.

After talking it over with Keith, I decided that I needed to pull back. I remembered the rule for overtraining syndrome of reducing to 50 percent of usual training for two weeks. I decided to cross-train by biking and rollerblading, focusing on core and knee exercises, and skipping a few runs. It was just over thirteen weeks until Berlin, so I felt I still had some flexibility in my training regime. The next week instead of doing the two-hour, twenty-minute run my regime called for, I did a slow forty-five-minute jog, covering only six kilometres.

Within a few days I noticed a big difference. I felt stronger, my cough was gone, my sinus pain resolved, and I was eager to get back on the program. I knew that pushing too hard too soon could wipe away the benefits I was feeling and most likely worsen my knee pain, so I kept holding back for the next few days.

JULY 5

This morning a patient asked me to refer him for medically assisted death. It was the first time I had had such a request, but I knew they would be coming as the Canadian Supreme Court had legalized this type of medical assistance in dying. The rules around such decisions require that the patient be suffering from intolerable physical or mental anguish and be capable of understanding their decision. My patient told me that his Parkinson's disease caused him intolerable suffering and that although his medications have been adjusted innumerable times, he continued to suffer and did not want to keep living. When I explored his feelings, he said he didn't want to have a painful or dramatic death but instead wanted to plan his death and let his family know so they could be prepared. I helped make the referral to the group of physicians who had started to work with patients to plan such decisions, and we agreed to meet again before he took any further steps.

I thought of him while I was out running tonight. The sun was just setting, and my wife and children were asleep. I passed groups of cyclists and ran along floodlit fields where young women were playing soccer. I ran through the dark wooded area of Vincent Massey Park and watched as fireflies punctuated the night. As I came out to the flat grass beyond the park, groups of bats swooped over me. It was humid and I was dripping with sweat by the time I tiptoed in through the back door. Inside, the air conditioning was flowing through the house. I drank two glasses of ice water, and felt my breathing and heart rate slow to normal. My eyelids grew heavy. What would tomorrow bring? I went to sleep.

JULY 13

Today was my longest run in three weeks. I was back on track with my training and I felt ready for the challenge. As I was finishing my clinic notes for that morning's patients, my wife texted me, "Please don't run for 2.5 hours in this heat, it's over 40°C with humidex. We'll find another time that works." She wasn't the only one warning me about the heat. As I passed through the office kitchen, my colleague Natasha warned me, "It's so hot out there it makes you nauseous." I had my CamelBak water bag and three energy gel packs. The heat would certainly slow me down, but I knew that if I didn't go today, then I wouldn't be ready to do my next and even longer run next week, and the Berlin Marathon clock said ten weeks and three days. It was time to step up.

I had a route planned that mostly involved shaded trails through parks and along the river shore, which I knew would be cooler. I started out slowly, feeling the humidity press against me. Within a few minutes my shirt was soaked so I took it off and carried it awkwardly rolled up in a ball in one hand. I saw the changing of the guards outside the Governor General's estate and could only imagine how hot the soldiers were, wearing traditional British red uniforms with tall black beefeaters hats. I climbed a hill overlooking the Ottawa River, then ran down the shore where a gravel path follows the river for over ten kilometres. In the early 1950s my mother would walk to this very part of the river from her home in Green's Creek on the edge of Ottawa as it was at that time. Her parents had met in London during the war then built their own home and a new life in Canada.

I ran slowly, pacing myself in the heat. As I headed back, the wind picked up and grey clouds race overhead. Suddenly, cool rain was pelting down. I stood at the shore of the river for a moment with my arms outstretched, feeling my body cool in the summer rain. A few minutes later the rain stopped. When I got back to my office, Melissa texted me, "Did you survive?" and my colleague Natasha smiled as she saw me stagger through the back door of the clinic, dripping in sweat and rain.

AUGUST 7

Seven weeks before Berlin I go for a run with my brother Sascha. He has come to Canada from England, where he lives with his wife, Angela. They are spending three weeks exploring Ontario and Quebec, and we have taken them to a favourite cottage of ours. Sascha and his wife get up and go running most mornings, exploring new trails while Melissa and I stay home and get the kids ready for the day. They discover a 3K route from the cottage that leads directly to the middle of the nearby beach.

Today Sascha offers to show me the route. We set out at 5:00 p.m., but it still feels like noon, with high humidity and a blazing sun. Sascha paces himself with his running watch. He tells me he will run slower than usual because the heat is raising his heart rate, but it is still a fast pace for me. Sascha has become a barefoot runner and has put a lot of thought into his form. As we run, Sascha encourages me to lean forward so my feet are never hitting the ground in front of me. He also encourages me to increase my cadence. We turn left and head through a small campground filled with RVs and tents before coming out along a small river that runs into Lake Ontario at the beach. The sun is low directly ahead of us and there are small waves lapping the shore.

We pause for less than a minute then turn back toward home. There is more uphill on the way back and we are both breathing harder. The pace remains quick, but I am leaning forward and I find it makes me feel faster. Running with Sascha is motivating me to push harder and I think about how much faster I could be if we trained together.

After he leaves, I read about ChiRunning, a style of running form articulated by Danny Dreyer that draws on tai chi. The tenets of ChiRunning are keeping your back straight but leaning forward slightly and focusing on midfoot strikes directly under the body. I ask Sascha if this is what inspired him, but he insists he has never heard of ChiRunning, but the form made sense for him and he has adopted it into his own style.

AUGUST 14

I think I've run more in the past week since we have been back from the cottage than ever before. Sixty-one kilometres. It sounds like a lot to me. But more importantly, I feel I've also run faster and felt better. Is this because of the relative rest at the cottage or because of the new techniques that Sascha encouraged me to try? I have been leaning forward a bit, I've been focusing on my core and on my foot strike.

On Monday I ran a relaxed forty-five minutes, then on Tuesday I ran for thirty minutes and did some core work in the park. Wednesday was a hot day with the humidex reaching 41°C. I filled my CamelBak to the brim and packed the last sports gel I had along with two little boxes of raisins and set out.

I had been reading Adharanand Finn's book *The Way of the Runner* for the past week and was just getting to the final chapters. I felt that I really knew Finn and could relate to his experience of struggling with improving his running form while at the same time finding his true motivation from a simple love of the experience of running itself. I had read before about the marathon monks and the practice of *Ekiden*, a distinctly Japanese type of relay race involving teams of varying sizes running varying distances usually in the 10–20K range.

After just over ten kilometres, I turned around still feeling strong. I ate my only gel. Around five kilometres from the end, I ran out of water in my CamelBak. It was the first time I'd gone through the full two litres on a run. I got back to my office and went straight into the pharmacy below, feeling the cold blast of air conditioning against my wet skin. I picked up a protein bar and a bottle of cold sparkling water, then sat down by the cash and drank and ate until I felt the strength returning to my legs. I still had to bike home, pick up the kids from school, and make dinner.

I took Thursday off from running, in part because I ended up working through lunch and in part because I felt I deserved the rest. On Friday I was scheduled for another one hour, fifty-minute run. I felt more tired than usual and wondered if I was up for another long run. It had been raining much of the day and I briefly imagined spending the night at home watching old episodes of *Star Trek* or going to bed early. In the end, I managed to set off at around 8:30 p.m., just after the kids went to sleep. I hadn't made it to the nearby cycling store that sells sports gels, so all I had was a Ziploc bag with five apricots. I remembered Dan carrying a little bag of apricots when we ran the trail race in May, so I was confident it would be enough.

Twenty minutes into the run, I felt the life flow back into my whole body. All the fatigue and stress of the day began to melt away. It was just me running through the cool night. The Pleiades were supposed to be raining down, but it was too cloudy to see any stars at all. Again I thought about my form, leaning forward, midfoot striking, staying in my zones. I felt good going fast and I followed the canal to the Ottawa River, then ran past Parliament Hill and through a series of tunnels under the roads. As I exited one tunnel, I heard the roar of a crowd and the drone of rock music as the path took me right behind the stage of an outdoor concert. "What's up, Ottawa?" the musician shouted to roars from the crowd.

I was buoyed by the energy of the night as I ran past the War Museum. After the museum, the lights on the path came to an end and I was running only by the glint of the half moon. I ran down a hill to a rail bridge that passes over the river toward Quebec. I clenched my fist as I realized I was at the halfway point. On the way back I again passed the concert then had to pick my way through groups of people walking along the canal late at night. I got home and within a few minutes I was falling into a very deep sleep.

Today is Sunday. It is the day of the women's Olympic marathon. I had an eighty-minute run today. My legs were tired, but I still managed to keep a good pace and felt strong afterward. As I was running,

I wondered if I'd get back in time to watch the final kilometres of the marathon. It was just after 10:30 when I reached home, so I turned on my computer and opened the live stream. It was kilometre thirty-nine and Jemima Sumgong was leading by a few steps. Sumgong maintained her lead and dashed through the ribbon nine seconds ahead of her competitor. I was surprised that it was Kenya's first gold in the Olympic women's marathon, although they had won silver in the past three Olympics.

AUGUST 21

The next week I am watching the men's Olympic marathon. It is a hot day in Rio and the race comes down to the three runners — Eliud Kipchoge, Feyisa Lilesa, and Galen Rupp. I watch most of the race while we get ready to host a brunch. Eliud is the clear favourite and has unstoppable form. Lilesa is a strong finisher in second place. The real surprise is seeing a native of Oregon beating a group of Kenyans and Ethiopians to take the bronze medal.

It is only afterward that I reflect on the motion Lilesa was making with his hands as he finished the race. He held his arms over his head to form a cross. I thought it some kind of victory symbol at the time and afterward learned it was a protest sign to bring attention to the Ethiopian government's treatment of the Oromo people. It is another chapter in the long history of athletes and nations using the Games to bring attention to their political struggles. It is incredibly effective as the eyes of the world gaze intently on the Games and the heroic athletes for only two weeks every four years.

AUGUST 31

Ten days later I take the morning off work to focus on my training run. At three hours, ten minutes, it will be my longest training run. It is a perfect morning, and I am eager to get moving. I drop my children at school, walk out of the schoolyard, and immediately start running. I have a route planned, but I don't know how far I will go. I follow the Ottawa River and go farther downriver than ever before. Cyclists methodically push past me going in both directions. I pass the city's water treatment plant, the federal Ministry of Health at Tunney's Pasture, and run on to the bridge to Quebec. I pass the sandy swath of the Westboro Beach and run on. I reach the halfway point and with a last glance toward the horizon, I turn back toward home.

The run home feels quicker. As I reach the 3:10 mark, I still feel good, so I break into a sprint. I envision myself passing through the Brandenburg Gate. I thrill at the speed. In the end I just break thirty kilometres. Is that right on track? Too slow? Whatever the pace, I now know I can do the distance. It is three weeks until Berlin, and I believe I can finish.

SEPTEMBER 25 – BERLIN MARATHON

This year the Berlin Marathon is held on Sunday, September 25. I come to the city two days before the race with my son. My father is also in Berlin, and he will watch Oliver during the race. Before I can relax, I need to pin my race number to my shirt and attach my timing chip to my shoes, so soon after arriving, we head over to the marathon centre, which is located in a former train station next to the Landwehr Canal.

Although my training was not perfect, it is over now. The next morning I go on a twenty-minute run to get my bearings, but other than the marathon, that is the only running I will do in Berlin. We spend the day exploring the city, taking Oliver to the zoo. It is a calm, thoughtful, ordered, playful city. I breathe in its eight hundred years of history for just a moment. Then it's race day.

It is early on Sunday and the streets are thick with runners. I hear an announcer declare that this year there are forty-one thousand participants from 122 countries. We stream toward the starting area through the Tiergarten. As I walk through the chill of the morning, I finish half of the *Einstein Kaffee* my father brought me. In old pictures of the city, you can see the Berlin Wall passing just metres in front of the entrance to the Tiergarten. After the Second World War, the British authorities turned areas of the park into vegetable gardens to feed starving Berliners. Many of the two hundred thousand trees were chopped down for firewood. Then, in the 1960s, the trees were replanted and over time the park grew back into a wild and verdant place of tranquility.

But today it is not tranquil as tech-clad athletes pick their way through the forest path to get to their starting zones. I arrive only about ten minutes before the start of the elite race, but I know it will take some time before the bulk of humanity starts to move. At 9:15 exactly, the starting gun goes. A few minutes later I feel a surge of excitement as we start shuffling forwards toward the start line. And then we are off. To pace myself, I am wearing an old Timex that belonged to my wife in high school. I start the timer, get to my race pace, and feel the cadence of the run take over my body as I find my form and mentally prepare for the longest run of my life.

The river of marathoners floods down Berlin's main streets. Lining the route are people of all ages cheering the runners on, urging them to push on through the pain, or yelling to their loved ones to *Lauf!* You find a rhythm running with a pack of marathoners. I am beautifully on pace. I feel happy, uplifted. I feel a great affection for the runners around me, for the crowds, for everyone. When I pass a rock band or a traditional German brass band or a group of drummers urging us on, I put my hands in the air, clap, and cheer. I feel exuberantly alive. I remember my patient saying that he never felt as exhilarated in his life as after finishing the marathon. I think about my son, my daughter, and my wife still asleep back in Ottawa. *This is what I came for. When this is over, I will be a marathoner.*

In my mind I have broken the race into four 10K blocks, with a 2K bonus at the end. We pass the 10K mark and I reset my watch and mentally gear up for the second quarter. We run over so many canals. I had read that there are more bridges in Berlin than in Venice. I was contemplating this at the 13K mark and gazing dreamily into the distance when I caught my foot on the top of a speed bump. I stumbled and lurched forward but managed to steady myself before I hit the ground. I settled back into my rhythm. Nothing hurt; I would keep going. We passed a huge mural of a hammer and sickle and a Soviet man and woman looking triumphantly into the distance. The street widened into Karl Marx Boulevard, a wide four-lane vestige of the Soviet era. We ran down this road from the past for four kilometres before turning into another shaded parkway. It was then I began to tire.

Everything above my legs felt great. Mentally, I was thrilling at the experience. *This is a marathon.* Every forty-five minutes I was taking a peanut butter energy gel, and I had water at almost every station. Nothing hurt, but I could not will my legs to keep up the pace and like a ship drifting toward an open harbour, I slowed as I neared the end of the race. It was almost noon, and every few minutes, we would pass a downed runner wrapped in reflective blankets, someone holding up their legs while a paramedic calmly assessed their status. At a massage station at the halfway point, runners lay on their stomachs while therapists frantically worked on their muscles. At one point, an ambulance nudged through the crowd to recover another victim of the race.

I looked for my son and my dad as I passed near our hotel, but I couldn't find them in the crowd. We turned the final corner, and I could see the Brandenburg Gate in the distance. This had been my goal for the past year, and I was about to pass the threshold. I was a few minutes off my goal, but I didn't care. *I will be a marathoner.* The music surged and I felt waves of exhilaration pass through me. I was covered in sweat, the salt was forming crusts on my face, I was sunburned, and both my feet were starting to hurt.

I crossed the finish line and stumbled a few metres. My legs felt like deadwood. Walking took immense effort. I felt a great thirst. My gaze drifted, and I heard the word *hypnagogic* in my mind — those transitional moments before sleep. Was I going to black out? *Thirsty.* I was so thirsty. A runner in front of me asked a paramedic if there was water and he pointed up and around the corner. It seemed so far away. We staggered in that direction. A woman wearing latex gloves handed me three figs. I bit into the dark fruit, trying to squeeze out the water. Once I made it to the drinks table, I was wary of hyponatremia, the medical condition of having too much water relative to salt in your blood, so I tried to limit my water intake. I wanted to get back to the hotel, but first I needed to rest. I found a patch of grass and lay down in the shade of a small tree. Runners were stumbling all around me. I didn't want to get up. After ten minutes I thought I would try; pulling myself up, I felt dull pain throughout both my calves.

Over the next thirty minutes I staggered home and found my son and dad waiting for me. I lay on the thick carpet of the hotel room. My wife called from Ottawa. "I was getting worried," she lamented from far away. I told her the story of the race, the glory and the pain.

I had promised my son we would go swimming after the marathon, so we went outside and saw the streams of runners continuing to flow toward the Brandenburg Gate. We took a taxi to a beautiful art deco public pool. The water was cold and refreshing. The pain in my legs ceased as I kicked and rolled through the water. I met another runner recovering in the pool and we compared notes. Later at the hotel sauna, I met Alexander, a Swedish businessman who had just run in Berlin for the third time. "Up until thirty kilometres, I was going for a personal best but then I hit the wall," he told me. His favourite course was Chicago and his local Stockholm Marathon was challenging because of the bridges and the elevation.

We left Berlin the next morning but not before interacting with dozens of runners of all nationalities. At forty-one thousand strong, we formed a city within a city. Many wore race jackets or finisher shirts; some wore medals over their dress clothes. Many walked strangely, limping in a range of gaits, testimony to a panoply of painful muscles and joints. Waiting to board our flight, everyone around me was reviewing their race pace and cadence on their phones, sharing stories with each other in a medley of European languages. We had finished what we started on the first day of training all those months ago, and now we could go home.

As we flew away from Berlin, I thought about the next race I had planned, my favourite 10K dash through Oka National Park just outside of Montreal. I thought about the next marathon — would it be London, Stockholm, Amsterdam? La Chute du Diable? How would I improve? Run more volume, train with more fast intervals, focus more on strengthening, possibly by working with a trainer at a little studio in my neighbourhood. That was in the future. Today I wouldn't run, but tomorrow, tomorrow I would start my new training plan with a gentle thirty-minute exploration of the Athens neighbourhood where I would be visiting my mother. My passion for running had ascended again to another level, like a rich marriage, where the longer I ran the deeper my love grew.

SEPTEMBER 28

Three days later I was on the island of Aegina, just across the bay from Athens. I stepped out of the quiet oasis of the Hotel Rastoni and jogged two minutes to the coastal road. In front of a temple dedicated to Aphrodite, I turned right and followed the ruins until the ocean opened up beside me. A white cat perching on top of a garbage bin looked up as I passed. The roar of a moped passed behind me. The sun was full as a cool breeze blew in from the sea. In the distance I saw the broad mountainous outline of mainland Greece. The day before, my son and I had climbed to the top of the Acropolis and looked out across the city toward the ocean. My legs felt stiff from the marathon, but every day was getting better. I passed a small lighthouse perched on a rocky outcropping. I picked up my pace and ran downhill past a small inlet choked with seaweed. There was ocean all around me. I remembered the rush of the marathon, the exhilaration. Tomorrow we would be going home. In five weeks I would be racing in Oka.

OCTOBER 12

It's been two weeks since Berlin, and I just ran my longest training run yet for Oka. It was a seventy-five-minute progression run to Parliament Hill and back. The canal had been drained of water overnight and I observed the debris of the past summer including two bicycles, some traffic bollards, and a variety of dead birds. It was a fast run, covering almost fourteen kilometres. It is unseasonably warm, much warmer than it has been for the past week.

But the days are getting shorter, and I've been talking to my patients about getting ready for possible seasonal affective disorder (SAD) symptoms as winter arrives. My colleague told me today, "I'm getting busy, everyone is coming in with mental health complaints early this year."

Last winter, so many people struggled with their mood, including my colleagues, friends and patients. I started advising use of SAD lights of 10,000 lux for at least thirty minutes per day to almost everyone.

NOVEMBER 6

Today was the New York City Marathon. Mary Keitany, whom I had seen run by my house a few years earlier, won for a third time. The male group saw the youngest winner in race history, an Eritrean named Ghirmay Ghebreslassie, who is only twenty years old. My dad was visiting New York and called to tell me about the spirit of running in the air. He said it reminded him of our time together in Berlin two months earlier.

At Oka, in a small national park on the shores of the Ottawa River, I ran the 10K race I had been training for since Berlin. I got to the start line only ten minutes before the race and joined the eight hundred other runners in a group warm-up led by a tall man with a long ponytail yelling instructions in French into his microphone. The early-morning sun diffracted through the forest and only a hundred metres in the distance was a widening of the Ottawa River called Lake of Two Mountains. This was my third time in Oka, and as soon as I walked to the start line, I felt a jolt of euphoria as I recalled my past races.

I started the race fast, checking my little Timex watch to ensure I was on pace. It was a bright and still morning in the forest. The only sound was my breathing. Every few minutes a group of runners would cluster together, but for much of the race I was on my own or pacing myself next to one or two other runners. The first hill started after three kilometres and there was a turnaround halfway up the hill just as we passed the 4K marker. The pace started to wear on me, but I kept pushing. After the halfway mark the kilometres seemed to get farther and farther apart. My mind played tricks on me, as a flash of yellow clothing or yellow leaves would look to me like the yellow kilometre markers placed along the course. Each time I climbed another hill, I was sure it was the last. I pushed through the final kilometre finishing within my goal, my breath coming short and fast. I walked a few metres to the recovery tent, picked up a banana and chocolate milk, and decided to head home.

With Oka behind me I had completed my races for the year — the half-marathon trail run in Wakefield, the Berlin Marathon, and now my victory lap in Oka. For next year, I had planned a winter half-marathon for February, another trail run, perhaps the half-marathon in

Mont Tremblant and a fall marathon. Of course, I would also return to Oka in November. I got an email from a running group urging me to "Make Next Year Your Best Running Year Yet." That was certainly the plan. I would keep focusing on my core strength, pushing my training pace, and figuring out hydration and nutrition during the long runs. I would work on avoiding injury and overtraining. Although I had been a runner since childhood, I was now five years into my second life as a runner. During this time, I had seen the birth of my two children, grown into my work as a physician, and woven running into the essential fabric of life. Would the next year be my best running year yet?

AFTERWORD

The human body was designed to run on the savannahs of a newly cooling African subcontinent and to carry the human brain, the source of our astoundingly complex techno-industrial civilization. We carry inside us vestiges of this ancient origin, and we suppress and ignore these relics of our old life at our own peril. As a scientist, I aspire to the purest state of rationality; I admire the incredible analytical power we can harness to solve problems and build our future. But this brain has also created a world of inactivity. Running washes us in sweat and rekindles our link to nature. When I sprint on a dirt trail tracing a wide river, I reach into my evolutionary past and feel the euphoria of putting my body to the use for which it was designed.

Running is also a privilege. To have the health, the time, the energy, the safety, and the will to run is not a given. I am particularly aware of this when running in Ottawa at night. I feel so safe and so serene, but I've seen enough of the world to know that being out at night is not safe for most people. There is a risk of crime and assault, and there is the also the risk of being injured by a car or motorcycle unless you have access to well-lit and protected paths. Even poor countries and poor neighbourhoods spend large portions of their budgets on road maintenance and safety, but creating safe recreational paths for walkers, runners, and cyclists is usually the last priority.

Taking time off work or away from family responsibilities to travel to races is also a privilege that was unheard of in human history. It has become extremely popular around the world, but entry fees and the need for gear such as proper clothing and shoes still pose a challenge to those with little disposable income. Running is a way of life and a path to greatness in countries such as Kenya and Ethiopia, but for every Eliud Kipchoge, there are hundreds if not thousands of young men and women who are unbelievably fast and hard-working but never make it to the front of the line or the international stage. Bad luck, injuries, and the needs of family or farm prevent many with great potential from fulfilling their early promise. Running is our common birthright as a species, but running is also a gift that must be cherished and shared through reducing barriers to entry and ensuring that those who need its benefits the most can use the sport to better themselves.

Fortunately, running is well-positioned to be a democratic pursuit. I have seen many people who would never dream of running make the decision to start with walking, begin to jog, begin to run, and then become passionate and regular runners. Nor is running only reserved for the fast, the lithe, and the lanky. People who take the time to slowly jog or walk a 10K or half-marathon are putting in many more hours on race day than the professionals who breeze through in a matter of minutes. And it's not necessary to run only to win races. Running can help you to socialize, to burn off stress, or to commute.

I've recently become "one of those guys" that you see in running gear with a backpack heading to the office. It's taken a while, but it was a natural next step in my running journey. I normally bike to work, but as the snow has fallen this winter, I have put away my bike and begun packing my work clothes into my backpack and taking off for work by foot. The first time it seemed like a novelty, although I've run the 6K distance hundreds of times before in training runs. It only took half an hour and I get to work feeling even better than before. Most days I also run at lunch or run home in the afternoon. Now that I've crossed this cognitive barrier, I don't understand what's been preventing me from doing this all along. I see people prevented from exercising because of cognitive barriers every day, but I've realized that once we cast them aside it's hard to remember why they ever held us back in the first place.

DECEMBER 7

Today I ran with a destination in mind. It was my first foray to a new coffee bar in the ByWard Market in Ottawa's downtown. I had heard they use a variety of brewing techniques including French press, siphon, Chemex, pour-over, and more recent technological innovations. My memory of running in Montreal in October was coffee and running, a perfect combination of heat, sweat, caffeine, and the calming void. Wet snow fell the whole morning as I picked my way along the canal path toward downtown. Ottawa's rush hour slid alongside me, but I barely noticed. I was intent on my destination.

My pace has slowed slightly in recent weeks. After my fast race in Oka, I haven't been able to convince myself that I need to be fast as I train for my next half-marathon, which is still three months away. The snow and ice, which began in earnest in recent weeks, have also slowed me down. One morning as I ran to work, the snow had fallen so heavily overnight that I was forced to jump up and out with each stride, as if running on a beach of deep sand. When I got to work, my colleague Betty asked if I had ever seen a moose running through deep snow — "It goes so fast, it's as if it's nothing," even with the snow up to its neck.

I arrived at the coffee bar in just over half an hour. The staff were exuberant and talkative. Sophie told me that she was born in England and moved around as her father was in the Canadian military. Louise, seeing my running garb, told me she had run the Toronto Marathon last year and was running her second marathon in Ottawa this coming May. I watched them prepare an array of different type of brews as the snow continued to fall outside on York Street. I savoured the experience. Sophie tested a French press she had just brewed and exclaimed, "There is so much flavour, it makes me salivate." I sipped three cups of coffee, each brewed differently. I felt so peaceful. I knew I had just discovered another way to enjoy running.

On my way home I focused on how soft it felt to run on the newly fallen snow. My legs felt so much better running in the winter. The other day I told my wife that the most comfortable article of clothing I own, by far, is my pair of running tights. I tried to explain how they always felt right. Even in the extremes of Canadian winter they felt warm — but they never felt too warm. I was self-conscious, but she smiled sympathetically and said she understood.

I ran over the Bank Street Bridge, which arches high over the canal. The sky was winter grey-blue. The year was almost over. I saw a play last week about a son coming to terms with the death of his father. When the undertaker came to collect his father's body, the son asked the man whether his job working with the dead had taught him about life. The undertaker replied that it had made him appreciate the little things more, like the feeling of rain. The actor closed his eyes and stretched out his hands on the dimly lit stage as if he were feeling rain. As I crossed over the bridge and the snow hit my face, this memory blended with that of one of my favourite passages in fiction, the ending of James Joyce's story "The Dead":

> Yes, the newspapers were right: snow was general all over Ireland … It was falling, too, upon every part of the lonely churchyard on the hill where Michael Furey lay buried. It lay thickly drifted on the crooked crosses and headstones, on the spears of the little gate, on the barren thorns. His soul swooned slowly as he heard the snow falling faintly through the universe and faintly falling, like the descent of their last end, upon all the living and the dead.

I turn off the bridge and onto the narrow canal path. I feel so alive. The ice shimmers on the bark of the maple trees. I can smell the winter. I am almost home. I will keep running, this year, next year. I will run on and on into the distance. I will run with my eyes open, reaching out, sharing my experience, holding the hands of my children, my family, my friends, feeling the rain.

ACKNOWLEDGEMENTS

This book, perhaps like all books about running, has been a labour of love. Everyone mentioned in this book who went running with me and who read earlier drafts — my friends, my brothers, Alex Hutchinson, Adharanand Finn, and many more helped make this book possible. My own patients inspire me every day with their examples of courage and resilience. I have changed all names and identifying details to protect their privacy. Ultimately, it took belief from my family, my editors at Dundurn, and my agent, Lloyd Kelly, to turn the original manuscript into this book. I again want to thank the whole team at Dundurn for their wisdom and professionalism.

NOTES

PREFACE

1 L.R. Callahan, "Overview of Running Injuries of the Lower Extremity," *UTDOL* 2016.

CHAPTER I: BEGINNING TO RUN

1 D.E. Lieberman and D.M. Bramble, "The Evolution of Marathon Running Capabilities in Humans," *Sports Medicine* 37, nos. 4–5 (2007): 288–90.

2 Lieberman and Bramble, 288.

3 I. Tattersall, *Masters of the Planet: The Search for Our Human Origins* (New York: Palgrave Macmillan, 2012), 43.

4 D.E. Lieberman, "Is Exercise Really Medicine? An Evolutionary Perspective," *Current Sports Medicine Reports* 14, no. 4 (July–August 2015): 313–19.

5 Lieberman and Bramble, 289.

6 Tattersall, 28.
7 Tattersall, 29.
8 Lieberman, D.E., *The Story of the Human Body: Evolution, Health, and Disease* (New York: Vintage Books, 2013), 36.
9 Tattersall, 33.
10 Tattersall, 33.
11 Howard Russell Tuttle, "Human Evolution," *Encyclopedia Britannica*, posted February 3, 2020, britannica.com/science/human-evolution.
12 Tuttle, "Human Evolution."
13 Lieberman, 68.
14 Tattersall, 49.
15 Tattersall, 36.
16 Tattersall, 37.
17 Tattersall, 91.
18 Tattersall, 91.
19 Tattersall, 94.
20 Mark P. Mattson, "Evolutionary Aspects of Human Exercise — Born to Run Purposefully," *Ageing Research Reviews* 11, no. 3 (July 2012): 347–52.
21 Lieberman and Bramble, 289.
22 T. Noakes and M. Spedding, "Olympics: Run for Your Life," *Nature* 487 (July 19, 2012): 295–96.
23 Lieberman, 97.
24 Lieberman, 84.
25 Lieberman, 85.
26 Lieberman and Bramble, 289.
27 Lieberman and Bramble, 289.
28 Noakes and Spedding, 296.
29 Lieberman D., "Human Locomotion and Heat Loss: An Evolutionary Perspective," *Comparative Physiology* 5, no. 1 (January 2015): 99–117.
30 Lieberman, 85.
31 Lieberman and Bramble, 345.
32 Noakes and Spedding, 296.
33 Lieberman, 81
34 Lieberman, 84.
35 Lieberman, 111.
36 Mattson, 348.

37 Mattson, 349.

38 D. Robson, "A Brief History of the Brain," *New Scientist* (September 21, 2011), newscientist.com/article/mg21128311-800-a-brief-history-of-the-brain/.

39 Noakes and Spedding, 296.

40 National Geographic Society, *Global Human Journey*, video, nationalgeographic.org/media/global-human-journey/.

41 S.B. Eaton, "An Evolutionary Perspective on Human Physical Activity: Implications for Health," *Comparative Biochemistry and Physiology* 136 (2003): 153–59.

42 Lieberman, 259.

43 Sylvia Kirchengast, "Physical Inactivity from the Viewpoint of Evolutionary Medicine," *Sports* 20, no. 2 (2014): 34–50.

44 S.B. Eaton, M. Shostack, and M. Konne, *The Paleolithic Prescription: A Program of Diet & Exercise and a Design for Living* (New York: Harper & Row, 1988).

45 Eaton, 157.

46 Kirchengast, 41.

47 Kirchengast, 41.

48 Kirchengast, 42.

49 Eaton, 157.

50 Eaton, 156.

51 Kirchengast, 42.

52 In Thor Gotaas, *Running: A Global History*, trans. Peter Graves (Chicago: University of Chicago Press, 2009), 85.

53 Gretchen Reynolds, *The First 20 Minutes: Surprising Science Reveals How We Can Exercise Better, Train Smarter, Live Longer*, (New York: Plume, 2013).

54 D. Peterson, "The Benefits and Risks of Exercise," *UTDOL* 2016.

55 F.W. Booth and S.J. Lees, "Fundamental Questions About Genes, Inactivity and Chronic Diseases," *Physiological Genomics* 28 (2007): 146–57.

56 Booth and Lees, 146.

57 In Booth and Lees, 146.

58 A. Murray and R.J.S. Costa, "Born to Run. Studying the Limits of Human Performance," *BMC Medicine* 10 (2012): 76.

59 Booth and Lees, 146.

60 Reynolds, 250.

61 J.Y. Chau et al., "Daily Sitting Time and All-Cause Mortality: A Meta-Analysis." *PLoS One* 8, no. 11 (2013): e8000.
62 Chau et al, 12.
63 Booth and Lees, 150.
64 Lieberman, 118.
65 Lieberman, 117.
66 Lieberman, 118.

CHAPTER II: RUNNING INTO MEDICINE AND SCIENCE

1 Reynolds, 101.
2 G.C. Rowe et al., "Running Forward: New Frontiers in Endurance Exercise Biology," *Circulation* 129, no. 7 (February 18, 2014): 798–810.
3 D.R. Bassett, J.R. Edward, and T. Howley, "Limiting Factors for Maximum Oxygen Uptake and Determinants of Endurance Performance," *Medicine & Science in Sports & Exercise* 32, no. 1 (January 2000): 70.
4 D. Systrom and G. Lewis, "Exercise Physiology," *UTDOL* 2014, accessed June 8, 2016.
5 Systrom and Lewis.
6 Systrom and Lewis.
7 Rowe et al., 802.
8 Mattson, 349.
9 Rowe et al., 802.

CHAPTER III: RUNNING AND PHYSICAL HEALTH

1 Kirchengast, 35.
2 R.M. Green, *A Translation of Galen's Hygiene: De Sanitate Tuenda* (Whitefish, MT: Literary Licensing, 2012).
3 Rowe et al, 806.
4 Peterson.
5 Peterson.
6 C. Fiuza-Luces et al., "Exercise Is the Real Polypill," *Physiology* 28, no. 5 (September 1, 2013): 330–58.
7 P.T. Williams, "Reduction in Incident Stroke Risk with Vigorous Physical Activity. Evidence from 7.7-Year Follow-up of the National Runners' Health Study," *Stroke* 40, no. 5 (May 2009): 1921–23.

8 Gotaas, 241.

9 Gotaas, 242.

10 Rowe et al., 798.

11 P. Schnohr, et al., "Dose of Jogging and Long-Term Mortality: The Copenhagen City Heart Study," *Journal of the American College of Cardiology* 65, no. 5 (February 10, 2015): 411–19.

12 Peterson.

13 Alex Hutchinson, *Which Comes First, Cardio or Weights?* (Toronto: McClelland & Stewart, 2011): 10.

14 Fiuza-Luces, 333.

15 D.C. Lee, C.J. Lavie, and R. Vedanthan, "Optimal Dose of Running for Longevity: Is More Better or Worse," *Journal of the American College of Cardiology* 65, no. 5 (2015): 420–22.

16 D.C. Lee, et al., "Leisure-Time Running Reduces All-Cause and Cardiovascular Mortality Risk," *Journal of the American College of Cardiology* 64 (2014): 472–81; 83.

17 Laura F. DeFina, "Athletes Performing Extraordinary Physical Activity (>10,000 MET Min/Week) at No Greater Risk of All-Cause or Cardiovascular-Disease Mortality," American Heart Association, conference abstract, 2019, abstractsonline.com/pp8/#!/7891/presentation/30918.

18 Schnohr et al., 414.

19 Lee et al. (2014), 475.

20 C.J. Lavie et al., "Effects of Running on Chronic Diseases and Cardiovascular and All-Cause Mortality," *Mayo Clinic Proceedings* (November 2015): 1541–52.

21 H.H. Kyu et al., "Physical Activity and Risk of Breast Cancer, Colon Cancer, Diabetes, Ischemic Heart Disease, and Ischemic Stroke Events: Systematic Review and Dose-Response Meta-Analysis for the Global Burden of Disease Study," *British Medical Journal* 354 (2016): i3857.

22 Haroon Siddique, "WHO's Recommended Level of Exercise Too Low to Beat Disease — Study," *The Guardian*, August 9, 2016, theguardian.com/science/2016/aug/09/whos-recommended-level-exercise-too-low-beat-disease-study.

23 K. Blond, et al., "Association of High Amounts of Physical Activity with Mortality Risk: A Systematic Review and Meta-Analysis," *British Journal of Sports Medicine* (August 12, 2019): 1195–1201.

24 J.C. Kerns et al., "Increased Physical Activity Associated with Less Weight Regain Six Years After 'The Biggest Loser' Competition," *Obesity* 25, no. 11 (November 2017): 1838–43.

25 Peterson.

26 Lavie et al., 1543.

27 Lieberman et al., "Knee Osteoarthritis Has Doubled in Prevalence Since the Mid-20th Century," *PNAS* (August 2017): doi.org/10.1073/pnas.1703856114.

28 Peterson.

29 Peterson.

30 K. Christensen et al., "Ageing Populations: The Challenges Ahead," *Lancet* 374, no. 9696 (October 3–9, 2009): 1196–1208.

31 S.G. Deeks, "HIV Infection, Inflammation, Immunosenescence and Aging," *Annual Review of Medicine* 62 (February 2011): 141–55.

32 E.H. Blackburn, "Telomere States and Cell Fates," *Nature* 408 (2000): 53–56.

33 M.A. Blasco, "Telomeres and Human Disease: Ageing, Cancer and Beyond," *Nature Reviews Genetics* 6 (2005): 611–22.

34 Reynolds, 245.

35 Hutchinson, 180.

36 Reynolds, 241.

37 P.D. Loprinzi and E. Sng, "Mode-Specific Physical Activity and Leukocyte Telomere Length Among U.S. Adults: Implications of Running on Cellular Aging," *Preventive Medicine* 85 (2016): 17–19.

38 Loprinzi and Sng.

39 Reynolds, 239.

40 Reynolds, 243.

41 Lisa Feldman Barrett, "How to Become a 'Superager,'" *New York Times*, Dec. 31, 2016.

42 Claire J. Steves, Mitul M. Mehta, Stephen H.D. Jackson, Tim D. Spector, "Kicking Back Cognitive Ageing: Leg Power Predicts Cognitive Ageing After Ten Years in Older Female Twins," *Gerontology* 62, no. 2 (2016):138–49, epub November 10, 2015.

43 Rod K. Dishman et al., "Neurobiology of Exercise," *Obesity* 14, no. 3 (March 2006): 345–56.

44 Mattson, 350.

CHAPTER IV: RUNNING AND MENTAL HEALTH

1 In Gotaas, 163.

2 Neal Bascomb, *The Perfect Mile: Three Athletes, One Goal, and Less Than Four Minutes to Achieve It* (Boston: Houghton Mifflin, 2004), 14.

3 J.H. O'Keefe et al., "Organic Fitness: Physical Activity Consistent with Our Hunter-Gatherer Heritage," *Physician and Sports Medicine* 38, no. 4 (December 2010): 11–18.

4 J.H. O'Keefe et al. (2010).

5 M.G. Berman, J. Jonides, and S. Kaplan. "The Cognitive Benefits of Interacting with Nature," *Psychological Science* 19, no. 12 (2008): 1207–12.

6 K.G. Baron et al., "Exercise to Improve Sleep in Insomnia: Exploration of the Bidirectional Effects," *Journal of Clinical Sleep Medicine* 9, no. 8 (August 15, 2013): 819–24.

7 In Hutchinson, 244.

8 S. Heijnen, B. Hommel, A. Kibele, and L.S. Colzato, "Neuromodulation of Aerobic Exercise — A Review," *Frontiers in Psychology* 6 (2015): 1890.

9 D.A. Raichlen et al., "Exercise-Induced Endocannabinoid Signaling Is Modulated by Intensity," *European Journal of Applied Physiology* 113, no. 4 (April 2013): 869–75.

10 E. Hoare, et al., "The Associations between Sedentary Behaviour and Mental Health among Adolescents: A Systematic Review," *International Journal of Behavioral Nutrition and Physical Activity* 13, no. 1 (October 8, 2016): 108.

11 F.B. Schulch et al., "Are Lower Levels of Cardiorespiratory Fitness Associated with Incident Depression? A Systematic Review of Prospective Cohort Studies," *Preventive Medicine* 93 (2016): 159–65.

12 Schulch et al.

13 Peterson.

14 Scott Douglas, *Running Is My Therapy: Relieve Stress and Anxiety, Fight Depression, Ditch Bad Habits, and Live Happier* (New York: The Experiment, 2018).

15 Reynolds, 198.

16 T.J. Schoenfeld et al., "Physical Exercise Prevents Stress-Induced Activation of Granule Neurons and Enhances Local Inhibitory Mechanisms in the Dentate Gyrus," *Journal of Neuroscience* 33, no. 18 (May 1, 2013): 7770–77.

17 Heijnen et al., 4.
18 Mattson, 350.
19 Mattson, 349.
20 S. Gradari et al., "Can Exercise Make You Smarter, Happier, and Have More Neurons? A Hormetic Perspective," *Frontiers in Neuroscience* 10 (2016): 93.
21 Reynolds, 207.
22 Douglas, 23.
23 Douglas, 26.
24 Gradari et al., 93.
25 Rowe et al., 804.
26 D.K. Ingram, "Age-Related Decline in Physical Activity: Generalization to Nonhumans," *Medicine & Science in Sports & Exercise* 32, no. 9 (September 2000): 1623–29.
27 B.N. Greenwood, A.B. Loughridge, N. Sadaoui, J.P. Christianson, and M. Fleshner, "The Protective Effects of Voluntary Exercise Against the Behavioral Consequences of Uncontrollable Stress Persist Despite an Increase in Anxiety Following Forced Cessation of Exercise," *Behavioural Brain Research* 233, no. 2 (2021): 314–21. doi.org/10.1016/j.bbr.2012.05.017.

CHAPTER V: RUNNING AND ADDICTION

1 Nora Volkow, "Running Helps Me Cope with Stress," posted March 19, 2012, YouTube video, youtube.com/watch?v=BYGX_0mUEKY.
2 B. Kaplan, "King of Pain," *iRun* 2 (2017).
3 Kaplan.
4 HOKA ONE ONE, "Women Who Fly: Catra Corbett," posted August 22, 2017, YouTube video, youtube.com/watch?v=GyaAtXkihtM.
5 A. Finn, *The Rise of the Ultra Runners: A Journey to the Edge of Human Endurance* (London: Guardian Faber, 2019), 105.
6 D. Wang et al., "Impact of Physical Exercise on Substance Abuse Disorders: A Meta-Analysis," *PLoS One* 9, no. 10 (2014): e110728.
7 Peterson.
8 M.S Buchowski et al., "Aerobic Exercise Training Reduces Cannabis Craving and Use in Non-Treatment Seeking Cannabis-Dependent Adults," *PLoS One* 6 (2011): e17465.

9 Esther Sophia Giesen and Wilhelm Bloch, "The Role of Exercise Therapy as a Complementary Measure in the Addiction Treatment of a Multiply Impaired Alcohol Dependent Client: A Case Report," *Journal of Substance Abuse & Alcoholism* 4, no. 1 (January 2016): jscimedcentral.com/SubstanceAbuse/substanceabuse-4-1041.pdf.

CHAPTER VI: RUNNING FASTER

1 Gotaas, 17.
2 Gotaas, 17.
3 Gotaas, 221.
4 Gotaas, 221.
5 J. Bale, "Kenyan Running Before the 1968 Mexico Olympics," in *East African Running Toward a Cross-Disciplinary Perspective*, ed. Y. Pitsiladis, J. Bale, C. Sharp, and T. Noakes (New York: Routledge, 2007).
6 E. Tam et al., "Energetics of Running in Top-Level Marathon Runners from Kenya," *European Journal of Applied Physiology* 112 (2012): 3797–806.
7 B. Saltin et al., "Aerobic Exercise Capacity at Sea Level and at Altitude in Kenyan Boys, Junior and Senior Runners Compared with Scandinavian Runners," *Scandinavian Journal of Medicine and Science in Sports* 5: 209–21.
8 B.W. Fudge et al., "Energy Balance and Body Composition of Elite Endurance Runners: A Hunter-Gatherer Phenotype," in *East African Running Toward a Cross-Disciplinary Perspective*, ed. Y. Pitsiladis, J. Bale, C. Sharp, and T. Noakes (New York: Routledge, 2007).
9 A. Finn, *Running with the Kenyans* (New York: Ballantine, 2012): 258.
10 Bascomb, 52.
11 Bascomb, 72.
12 Bascomb, 144.
13 Reynolds, 109.
14 Hutchinson, 235.
15 Hutchinson, 81.
16 Hutchinson, 100.
17 Hutchinson, 100.
18 Reynolds, 144.
19 Hutchinson, 106.

20 Reynolds, 132.
21 Hutchinson, 140.
22 Reynolds, 10.
23 Hutchinson, 123.
24 Hutchinson, 125.
25 Reynolds, 39.
26 Reynolds, 40.
27 Callahan.
28 Reynolds, 55.
29 Reynolds, 67.
30 Hutchinson, 90.
31 Bascomb, 118.

CHAPTER VII: RUNNING HURTS

1 Callahan.
2 Callahan.
3 Callahan.
4 Reynolds, 170.
5 K. Khan and A. Scott, "Overview of the Management of Overuse (Chronic) Tendinopathy," *UTDOL* 2017.
6 K.L. Maughan and B.R. Boggess, "Achilles Tendinopathy and Tendon Rupture," *UTDOL* 2015.
7 Callahan.
8 F.G. O'Connor and S.W. Mulvaney, "Patellofemoral Pain Syndrome," *UTDOL* 2016.
9 O'Connor and Mulvaney.
10 Callahan.
11 Hutchinson, 37.
12 Callahan.
13 D.E. Lieberman et al., "Foot Strike Patterns and Collision Forces in Habitually Barefoot versus Shod Runners," *Nature* 463 (January 28, 2010): 531–35.
14 Lieberman et al., 531.
15 Lieberman et al., 533.
16 O'Connor and Mulvaney.
17 A.R. Altman and I.S. Davis, "Prospective Comparison of Running

Injuries between Shod and Barefoot Runners," *British Journal of Sports Medicine* 50, no. 8 (April 2015): 476–80, epub June 30, 2015.

18 Callahan.

19 J.T. Fuller, et al., "Body Mass and Weekly Training Distance Influence the Pain and Injuries Experienced by Runners Using Minimalist Shoes: A Randomized Controlled Trial," *American Journal of Sports Medicine* 45, no. 2 (2017): 1162.

20 Callahan.

21 Reynolds, 164.

22 Aamer Madhani, "Treadmill Injuries Send Thousands to the ER Every Year," *USA Today*, May 4, 2015, usatoday.com/story/news/2015/05/04/treadmill-emergency-room-injuries-exercise-equipment/26898487/.

23 Hutchinson, 86.

24 Thomas M. Howard, "Overtraining Syndrome in Athletes," *UTDOL* (2015), uptodate.com/contents/overtraining-syndrome-in-athletes.

25 Howard.

26 C.A. Jaworski and D.B. Pyne, "Upper Respiratory Tract Infections: Considerations in Adolescent and Adult Athletes," *UTDOL* (2016), uptodate.com/contents/upper-respiratory-tract-infections .

27 Jaworski and Pyne.

28 Callahan.

29 Callahan.

30 Callahan.

CHAPTER VIII: RUNNING A MARATHON

1 C.N. DeWall, "How to Run Across the Country Faster Than Anyone," *New York Times*, October 26, 2016.

2 Gotaas, 40.

3 Gotaas, 131.

4 Gotaas, 135.

5 Gotaas, 137.

6 Gotaas, 137.

7 Gotaas, 139.

8 T. Ataide-Silva et al., "CHO Mouth Rinse Ameliorates Neuromuscular Response with Lower Endogenous CHO Stores," *Medicine & Science in Sports & Exercise*, epub April 29, 2016.

BIBLIOGRAPHY

Altman, A.R., and I.S. Davis. "Prospective Comparison of Running Injuries Between Shod and Barefoot Runners." *British Journal of Sports Medicine* 50, no. 8 (April 2015): 476–80. Epub June 30, 2015.

Ataide-Silva, T., Thaysa Ghiarone, Romulo Bertuzzi, Christos George Stathis, Carol Góis Leandro, Adriano Eduardo Lima-Silva. "CHO Mouth Rinse Ameliorates Neuromuscular Response with Lower Endogenous CHO Stores." *Medicine & Science in Sports & Exercise*. Epub April 29, 2016.

Bannister, Roger. *Twin Tracks*. London: Robson Press, 2014.

Baron K.G., Kathryn J. Reid, and Phyllis C. Zee. "Exercise to Improve Sleep in Insomnia: Exploration of the Bidirectional Effects." *Journal of Clinical Sleep Medicine* 9, no. 8 (August 15, 2013): 819–24.

Barrett, Lisa Feldman. "How to Become a 'Superager.'" *New York Times*, Dec. 31, 2016.

Bascomb, Neal. *The Perfect Mile: Three Athletes, One Goal, and Less Than Four Minutes to Achieve It*. Boston: Houghton Mifflin, 2004.

Bassett, D.R., J.R. Edward, and T. Howley. "Limiting Factors for Maximum Oxygen Uptake and Determinants of Endurance Performance." *Medicine & Science in Sports & Exercise* 32, no. 1 (January 2000): 70.

Berman, M.G., J. Jonides, and S. Kaplan. "The Cognitive Benefits of Interacting with Nature." *Psychological Science* 19, no. 12 (2008): 1207–12.

Blackburn, E.H. "Telomere States and Cell Fates." *Nature* 408 (2000): 53–56.

Blasco, M.A. "Telomeres and Human Disease: Ageing, Cancer and Beyond." *Nature Reviews Genetics* 6 (2005): 611–22.

Blond, K., C.F. Brinkløv, M. Ried-Larsen, A. Crippa, and A. Grøntved. "Association of High Amounts of Physical Activity with Mortality Risk: A Systematic Review and Meta-Analysis." *British Journal of Sports Medicine* (August 12, 2019): 1195–1201.

Booth, F.W., and S.J. Lees. "Fundamental Questions about Genes, Inactivity and Chronic Diseases." *Physiological Genomics* 28 (2007): 146–57.

Bramble, D.M., and D. Lieberman. "Endurance Running and the Evolution of *Homo*." *Nature* 432 (2004): 345–52.

Buchowski, M.S., Natalie N. Meade, Evonne Charboneau, Sohee Park, Mary S. Dietrich, Ronald L. Cowan, Peter R. Martin. "Aerobic Exercise Training Reduces Cannabis Craving and Use in Non-Treatment Seeking Cannabis-Dependent Adults." *PLoS One* 6 (2011): e17465.

Callahan, L.R. "Overview of Running Injuries of the Lower Extremity." *UTDOL* 2016.

Chau J.Y., Anne C. Grunseit, Tien Chey, Emmanuel Stamatakis, Wendy J. Brown, Charles E. Matthews, Adrian E. Bauman, and Hidde P. van der Ploeg. "Daily Sitting Time and All-Cause Mortality: A Meta-Analysis." *PLoS ONE* 8, no. 11 (2013): e8000.

Christensen, K., G. Doblhammer, R. Rau, and J.W. Vaupel. "Ageing Populations: The Challenges Ahead." *Lancet* 374, no. 9696 (October 3–9, 2009): 1196–1208.

Dawkins, Richard. *The Ancestor's Tale: A Pilgrimage to the Dawn of Evolution.* Boston: Houghton Mifflin Harcourt, 2004.

Deeks, S.G. "HIV Infection, Inflammation, Immunosenescence and Aging." *Annual Review of Medicine* 62 (February 2011): 141–55.

DeFina, Laura F. "Athletes Performing Extraordinary Physical Activity (>10,000

MET Min/Week) at No Greater Risk of All-Cause or Cardiovascular-Disease Mortality." Abstract. American Heart Association Conference (2019). abstractsonline.com/pp8/#!/7891/presentation/30918.

DeWall, C.N. "How to Run Across the Country Faster Than Anyone." *New York Times*, Oct. 26, 2016.

Dishman, Rod K., Hans-Rudolf Berthoud, Frank W. Booth, Carl W. Cotman, V. Reggie Edgerton, Monika R. Fleshner, Simon C. Gandevia, Fernando Gomez-Pinilla, Benjamin N. Greenwood, Charles H. Hillman, Arthur F. Kramer, Barry E. Levin, Timothy H. Moran, Amelia A. Russo-Neustadt, John D. Salamone, Jacqueline D. Van Hoomissen, Charles E. Wade, David A. York, Michael J. Zigmond. "Neurobiology of Exercise." *Obesity* 14, no. 3 (March 2006): 345–56.

Douglas, Scott. *Running Is My Therapy: Relieve Stress and Anxiety, Fight Depression, Ditch Bad Habits, and Live Happier.* New York: The Experiment, 2018.

Eaton, S.B. "An Evolutionary Perspective on Human Physical Activity: Implications for Health." *Comparative Biochemistry and Physiology* 136 (2003): 153–59.

Eaton, S.B., M. Shostack, and M. Konne. *The Paleolithic Prescription: A Program of Diet & Exercise and a Design for Living.* New York: Harper & Row, 1988.

Finn, Adharanand. *The Rise of the Ultra Runners: A Journey to the Edge of Human Endurance.* London: Guardian Faber, 2019.

———. *Running with the Kenyans.* New York: Ballantine, 2012.

Fiuza-Luces, C., Nuria Garatachea, Nathan A. Berger, Alejandro Lucia. "Exercise Is the Real Polypill." *Physiology* 28, no. 5 (September 1, 2013): 330–58.

Fudge, Barry W., Bengt Kayser, Klaas R. Westerterp, and Yannis Pitsiladis. "Energy Balance and Body Composition of Elite Endurance Runners: A Hunter-Gatherer Phenotype." In *East African Running Toward a Cross-Disciplinary Perspective*, edited by Yannis Pitsiladis, John Bale, Craig Sharp, and Timothy Noakes, 85–101. New York: Routledge, 2007.

Fuller, J.T., D. Thewlis, J.D. Buckley, N.A. Brown, J. Tsiros Hamill. "Body Mass and Weekly Training Distance Influence the Pain and Injuries Experienced by Runners Using Minimalist Shoes: A Randomized Controlled Trial." *American Journal of Sports Medicine* 45, no. 2 (2017): 1162.

Giesen, Esther Sophia, and Wilhelm Bloch. "The Role of Exercise Therapy as a Complementary Measure in the Addiction Treatment of a Multiply Impaired Alcohol Dependent Client: A Case Report," *Journal of Substance Abuse & Alcoholism* 4, no. 1 (January 2016): jscimedcentral.com/SubstanceAbuse/substanceabuse-4-1041.pdf.

Gotaas, Thor. *Running: A Global History*. Translated by Peter Graves. Chicago: University of Chicago Press, 2009.

Gradari, S., Anna Pallé, Kerry R. McGreevy, Ángela Fontán-Lozano, José L. Trejo. "Can Exercise Make You Smarter, Happier, and Have More Neurons? A Hormetic Perspective." *Frontiers in Neuroscience* 10 (2016): 93.

Green R.M. *A Translation of Galen's Hygiene: De Sanitate Tuenda.* Whitefish, MT: Literary Licensing, 2012.

Greenwood, B.N., A.B. Loughridge, N. Sadaoui, J.P. Christianson, and M. Fleshner. "The Protective Effects of Voluntary Exercise Against the Behavioral Consequences of Uncontrollable Stress Persist Despite an Increase in Anxiety Following Forced Cessation of Exercise." *Behavioural Brain Research* 233, no. 2 (2021): 314–21.

Heijnen, S., B. Hommel, A. Kibele, and L.S. Colzato. "Neuromodulation of Aerobic Exercise — A Review." *Frontiers in Psychology* 6 (2015): 1890.

Hoare, E., K. Milton, C. Foster, and S. Allender. "The Associations Between Sedentary Behaviour and Mental Health Among Adolescents: A Systematic Review." *International Journal of Behavioral Nutrition and Physical Activity* 13, no. 1 (October 8, 2016): 108.

HOKA ONE ONE. "Women Who Fly: Catra Corbett." Posted on August 22, 2017. YouTube video, 2:10, youtube.com/watch?v=GyaAtXkihtM.

Howard, Thomas M. "Overtraining Syndrome in Athletes." *UTDOL* 2015, uptodate.com/contents/overtraining-syndrome-in-athletes.

Hutchinson, Alex. *Which Comes First, Cardio or Weights?* Toronto: McClelland & Stewart, 2011.

Ingram, D.K. "Age-Related Decline in Physical Activity: Generalization to Nonhumans." *Medicine & Science in Sports & Exercise* 32, no. 9 (September 2000): 1623–29.

Jackson, Jonathan. "Iliotibial Band Syndrome." *UTDOL* 2016. Accessed February 12, 2017.

Jaworski, C.A., and D.B. Pyne. "Upper Respiratory Tract Infections: Considerations in Adolescent and Adult Athletes." *UTDOL* 2016, uptodate.com/contents/upper-respiratory-tract-infections.

Kaplan, B. "King of Pain," *iRun* 2 (2017).

Kerns, J.C., Juen Guo, Erin Fothergill, Lilian Howard, Nicolas D. Knuth, Robert Brychta, Kong Y. Chen, Monica C. Skarulis, Peter J. Walter, and Kevin D. Hall. "Increased Physical Activity Associated with Less Weight Regain Six Years After 'The Biggest Loser' Competition." *Obesity* 25, no. 11 (November 2017): 1838–43.

Khan, K., and A. Scott. "Overview of the Management of Overuse (Chronic) Tendinopathy." *UTDOL* 2017.

Kirchengast, Sylvia. "Physical Inactivity from the Viewpoint of Evolutionary Medicine." *Sports* 20, no. 2 (2014): 34–50.

Kyu, H.H., Victoria F. Bachman, Lily T. Alexander, John Everett Mumford, Ashkan Afshin, Kara Estep, J. Lennert Veerman, Kristen Delwiche, Marissa L. Iannarone, Madeline L. Moyer, Kelly Cercy, Theo Vos, Christopher J.L. Murray, and Mohammad H. Forouzanfar. "Physical Activity and Risk of Breast Cancer, Colon Cancer, Diabetes, Ischemic Heart Disease, and Ischemic Stroke Events: Systematic Review and Dose-Response Meta-Analysis for the Global Burden of Disease Study." *British Medical Journal* 354 (2016): i3857.

Lavie, C.J., Duck-chul Lee, Xuemei Sui, Ross Arena, James H. O'Keefe, Timothy S. Church, Richard V. Milani, and Steven N. Blair. "Effects of Running on Chronic Diseases and Cardiovascular and All-Cause Mortality." *Mayo Clinic Proceedings* (November 2015): 1541–52.

Lee, D.C., C.J. Lavie, and R. Vedanthan. "Optimal Dose of Running for Longevity: Is More Better or Worse." *Journal of the American College of Cardiology* 65, no. 5 (2015): 420–22.

Lee, D.C., R.R. Pate, C.J. Lavie, X. Sui, T.S. Church, and S.N. Blair. "Leisure-Time Running Reduces All-Cause and Cardiovascular Mortality Risk." *Journal of the American College of Cardiology* 64 (2014): 472–81.

Lee, I.M., E.J. Shiroma, F. Lobelo, P. Puska, S.N. Blair, and P.T. Katzmarzyk. "Effect of Physical Inactivity on Major Non-Communicable Diseases Worldwide: An Analysis of Burden of Disease and Life Expectancy." *Lancet* 380 (2012): 219–29.

Lieberman, D. "Human Locomotion and Heat Loss: An Evolutionary Perspective." *Comparative Physiology* 5, no. 1 (January 2015): 99–117.

Lieberman, D.E. "Is Exercise Really Medicine? An Evolutionary Perspective." *Current Sports Medicine Reports* 14, no. 4 (July–August 2015): 313–19.

Lieberman, D.E. *The Story of the Human Body: Evolution, Health, and Disease.* Vintage Books: New York, 2013.

Lieberman, D.E., and D.M. Bramble. "The Evolution of Marathon Running Capabilities in Humans." *Sports Medicine* 37, nos. 4–5 (2007): 288–90.

Lieberman, D.E., Ian J. Wallace, Steven Worthington, David T. Felson, Robert D. Jurmain, Kimberly T. Wren, Heli Maijanen, and Robert J. Woods. "Knee Osteoarthritis Has Doubled in Prevalence Since the Mid-20th Century." *PNAS* (August 2017). doi.org/10.1073/pnas.1703856114.

Lieberman D.E., Madhusudhan Venkadesan, William A. Werbel, Adam I. Daoud, Susan D'Andrea, Irene S. Davis, Robert Ojiambo Mang'Eni, and Yannis Pitsiladis. "Foot Strike Patterns and Collision Forces in Habitually Barefoot Versus Shod Runners." *Nature* 463 (January 28, 2010): 531–35.

Loprinzi, P.D., and E. Sng. "Mode-Specific Physical Activity and Leukocyte Telomere Length among U.S. Adults: Implications of Running on Cellular Aging." *Preventive Medicine* 85 (2016): 17–19.

Lutz, W., W. Sanderson, and S. Scherbov. "The Coming Acceleration of Global Population Aging." *Nature* 451 (2008): 716–19.

Madhani, Aamer. "Treadmill Injuries Send Thousands to the ER Every Year." *USA Today*, May 4, 2015, usatoday.com/story/news/2015/05/04/treadmill-emergency-room-injuries-exercise-equipment/26898487/.

Mattson, Mark P. "Evolutionary Aspects of Human Exercise — Born to Run Purposefully." *Ageing Research Reviews* 11, no. 3 (July 2012): 347–52.

Maughan, K.L., and B.R. Boggess. "Achilles Tendinopathy and Tendon Rupture." *UTDOL* 2015.

Möhlenkamp, Stefan, and Martin Halle. "Myocardial Adaptation in Response to Marathon Training: Do Short-Term Benefits Translate into Long-Term Prognosis?" *Circulation: Cardiovascular Imaging* 8 (2015): e003030.

Murray, Andrew, and Ricardo J.S. Costa. "Born to Run. Studying the Limits of Human Performance." *BMC Medicine* 10 (2012): 76.

National Geographic Society. *Global Human Journey*. Video. National Geographic Society. Accessed December 2, 2016. nationalgeographic.org/media/global-human-journey/.

Noakes T., and M. Spedding. "Olympics: Run for Your Life." *Nature* 487 (July 19, 2012): 295–96.

O'Connor, F.G., and S.W. Mulvaney. "Patellofemoral Pain Syndrome." *UTDOL* 2016.

O'Keefe J.H., B. Franklin, and C.J. Lavie. "Exercising for Health and Longevity vs Peak Performance: Different Regimens for Different Goals." *Mayo Clinic Proceedings* 89, no. 9 (September 1, 2014): 1171–75.

O'Keefe, J.H., C.J. Lavie, and M. Guazzi. "Part 1: Potential Dangers of Extreme Endurance Exercise: How Much Is Too Much? Part 2: Screening of School-Age Athletes." *Progress in Cardiovascular Diseases* 57 (2015): 396–405.

O'Keefe J.H., Robert Vogel, Carl J. Lavie, and Loren Cordain. "Organic Fitness: Physical Activity Consistent with our Hunter-Gatherer Heritage." *Physician and Sports Medicine* 38, no. 4 (December 2010): 11–18.

Pearson, Aria. "Out-of-Africa Migration Selected Novelty-Seeking Genes." *New Scientist* May 4, 2011. newscientist.com/article/mg21028114-400-out-of-africa-migration-selected-novelty-seeking-genes/.

Peterson, D. "The Benefits and Risks of Exercise." *UTDOL* 2016.

Pitsiladis, Yannis, John Bale, Craig Sharp, and Timothy Noakes, eds. *East African Running Toward a Cross-Disciplinary Perspective*. New York: Routledge: 2007.

Raichlen, D.A., A.D. Foster, A. Seillier, A. Giuffrida, and G.L. Gerdeman. "Exercise-Induced Endocannabinoid Signaling Is Modulated by Intensity." *European Journal of Applied Physiology* 113, no. 4 (April 2013): 869–75.

Rawson, R.A., Joy Chudzynski, Rachel Gonzales, Larissa Mooney, Daniel Dickerson, Alfonso Ang, Brett Dolezal, and Christopher B. Cooper. "The Impact of Exercise on Depression and Anxiety Symptoms Among Abstinent Methamphetamine-Dependent Individuals in A Residential Treatment Setting." *Journal of Substance Abuse Treatment* 57 (October 2015): 36–40.

Redelmeier, D., and J.A. Greenwald. "Competing Risks of Mortality with Marathons: Retrospective Analysis." *British Medical Journal* 335 (2007): 1275.

Reynolds, Gretchen. *The First 20 Minutes: Surprising Science Reveals How We Can Exercise Better, Train Smarter, Live Longer*. New York: Plume, 2013.

Robson, D. "A Brief History of the Brain." *New Scientist* (September 21, 2011). newscientist.com/article/mg21128311-800-a-brief-history-of-the-brain/.

Rodriguez, N.R., N.M. Di Marco, S. Langley, American Dietetic Association, Dietitians of Canada, American College of Sports Medicine. "Position of the American Dietetic Association, Dietitians of Canada, and the American College of Sports Medicine: Nutrition and Athletic Performance." *Medicine & Science in Sports & Exercise* 41, no. 3 (2009): 709.

Rowe, G.C., Adeel Safdar, Zolt Arany. "Running Forward: New Frontiers in Endurance Exercise Biology." *Circulation* 129, no. 7 (February 18, 2014): 798–810.

Sands, R.R. "Homo Cursor: Running into the Pleistocene." In *Anthropology of Sport and Human Movement: A Biocultural Perspective*, edited by Robert R. Sands and Linda R. Sands. Washington, D.C.: Lexington Books, 2012.

Schnohr, P., J.H. O'Keefe, J.L. Marott, P. Lange, and G.B. Jensen. "Dose of Jogging and Long-Term Mortality: The Copenhagen City Heart Study." *Journal of the American College of Cardiology* 65, no. 5 (February 10, 2015): 411–19.

Schoenfeld, T.J., Pedro Rada, Pedro R. Pieruzzini, Brian Hsueh, and Elizabeth Gould. "Physical Exercise Prevents Stress-Induced Activation of Granule Neurons and Enhances Local Inhibitory Mechanisms in the Dentate Gyrus." *Journal of Neuroscience* 33, no. 18 (May 1, 2013): 7770–77.

Schuch, F., D. Vancampfort, X. Sui, S. Rosenbaum, J. Firth, J. Richards, P. Ward, B. Stubbs. "Are Lower Levels of Cardiorespiratory Fitness Associated with Incident Depression? A Systematic Review of Prospective Cohort Studies." *Preventive Medicine* 93 (2016): 159–65.

Siddique, Haroon. "WHO's Recommended Level of Exercise Too Low to Beat Disease — Study." *Guardian*, August 9, 2016. theguardian.com/science/2016/aug/09/whos-recommended-level-exercise-too-low-beat-disease-study.

Sleiman, S., Jeffrey Henry, Rami Al-Haddad, Lauretta El Hayek, Edwina Abou Haidar, Thomas Stringer, Devyani Ulja, Saravanan S. Karuppagounder, Edward B. Holson, Rajiv R. Ratan, Ipe Ninan, and Moses V. Chao.

"Exercise Promotes the Expression of Brain Derived Neurotrophic Factor (BDNF) Through the Action of the Ketone Body β-Hydroxybutyrate." eLife (2016). doi: 10.7554/eLife.15092.

Steves, Claire J., Mitul M. Mehta, Stephen H.D. Jackson, and Tim D. Spector. "Kicking Back Cognitive Ageing: Leg Power Predicts Cognitive Ageing After Ten Years in Older Female Twins." *Gerontology* 62, no. 2 (2016):138–49. Epub November 10, 2015.

Systrom, D., and G. Lewis. "Exercise Physiology." *UTDOL* 2014. Accessed June 8, 2016.

Tam, E., Huber Rossi, Christian Moia, Claudio Berardelli, Gabriele Rosa, Carlo Capelli, and Guido Ferretti. "Energetics of Running in Top-Level Marathon Runners from Kenya." *European Journal of Applied Physiology* 112 (2012): 3797–806.

Tattersall, I. *Masters of the Planet: The Search for Our Human Origins.* New York: Palgrave Macmillan, 2012.

Trivedi, M.H., Tracy L. Greer, Chad D. Rethorst, Thomas Carmody, Bruce D. Grannemann, Robrina Walker, Diane Warden, Kathy Shores-Wilson, Mark Stoutenberg, Neal Oden, Meredith Silverstein, Candace Hodgkins, Lee Love, Cindy Seamans, Angela Stotts, Trey Causey, Regina P. Szucs-Reed, Paul Rinaldi, Hugh Myrick, Michele Straus, David Liu, Robert Lindblad, Timothy Church, Steven N. Blair, and Edward V Nunes. "Randomized Controlled Trial Comparing Exercise to Health Education for Stimulant Use Disorder: Results From the CTN-0037 Stimulant Reduction Intervention Using Dosed Exercise (STRIDE) Study." *Journal of Clinical Psychiatry* 78, no. 8 (2017): 1075–82.

Tuttle, Howard Russell. "Human Evolution." *Encyclopedia Britannica.* Posted February 3, 2020. britannica.com/science/human-evolution.

van der Wall, E.E. "Long-Distance Running: Running for a Long Life?" *Netherlands Heart Journal* 22, no. 3 (March 2014): 89–90.

van Mechelen, W., H. Hlobil, H.C. Kemper, W.J. Voorn, and H.R. de Jongh. "Prevention of Running Injuries by Warm-up, Cool-down, and Stretching Exercises." *American Journal of Sports Medicine* 21, no. 5 (1993): 71.

Volkow, Nora. "Running Helps Me Cope with Stress." Posted March 19, 2012. YouTube video, 2:05, youtube.com/watch?v=BYGX_0mUEKY.

Wallace, I.J. "Knee Osteoarthritis Has Doubled in Prevalence Since the Mid-20th Century." Proceedings of the National Academy of Sciences114, no. 35 (August 29, 2017): 9332–36.

Wang, D. Yanqiu Wang, Yingying Wang, Rena Li, and Chenglin Zhou. "Impact of Physical Exercise on Substance Use Disorders: A Meta-Analysis." *PLoS One* 9, no. 10 (2014): e110728.

Williams, P.T. "Reduction in Incident Stroke Risk with Vigorous Physical Activity. Evidence from 7.7-Year Follow-up of the National Runners' Health Study." *Stroke* 40, no. 5 (May 2009): 1921–23.

Wilson, E.O. *Consilience: The Unity of Knowledge*. New York: Vintage, 1998.

INDEX